# Konrad Kellen

## Reflections on Gluttony

### Edited by Dr. Bernd A. Weil

# Konrad Kellen

# REFLECTIONS ON GLUTTONY

## Understanding it and Dissolving it

**Edited by**

**Dr. Bernd A. Weil (PhD)**

## IMPRINT / IMPRESSUM

### Reflections on Gluttony

Original version

All rights: © Konrad Kellen (USA)

Alle Rechte liegen beim Autor.

Verleger und Herausgeber: Dr. phil. Bernd A. Weil (Germany)

Layout: Dr. Bernd Weil (Internet: www.bweil.de)

Production: Books on Demand GmbH

Printed in Germany

ISBN: 3-8311-1893-0

## Über den Autor Konrad Kellen (USA)

Konrad Katzenellenbogen, so hieß Konrad Kellen, bevor er die amerikanische Staatsbürgerschaft annahm, wurde am 14. Dezember 1913 in Berlin geboren und wuchs dort als Kind einer wohlhabenden deutsch-jüdischen Industriellenfamilie auf. Bereits während seines Jura–Studiums in München 1932 bekam Kellen die bedrohliche Nazi-Hetze und den fanatisch-patriotischen Hass der Ultra-Rechten zu spüren. Nach Hitlers Regierungsübernahme musste Kellen im März 1933 das ihm unerträglich gewordene Deutschland verlassen.

Mit Gelegenheitsarbeiten schlug er sich in Frankreich, den Niederlanden und Jugoslawien durch. 1935 gelangte er nach New York, später nach Los Angeles und wurde schließlich amerikanischer Staatsbürger. Von 1941 bis 1943 war Konrad Kellen Thomas Manns Privatsekretär im kalifornischen Pacific Palisades. "Konny", wie der "Zauberer" ihn nannte, tippte in dieser Zeit unter anderem Thomas Manns Manuskript "Joseph, der Ernährer" in die Maschine.

Kellen nahm als amerikanischer Offizier der "Psychologischen Kriegsführung" am Zweiten Weltkrieg teil, wurde ausgezeichnet und wirkte anschließend als Besatzungsoffizier in Deutschland bei der "Entnazifizierung" mit.

Nach der Rückkehr in die USA war Kellen 23 Jahre lang Mitglied der "Rand Corporation" (Santa Monica, CA), der berühmten amerikanischen "Denkfabrik".

Heute lebt Konrad Kellen mit seiner Ehefrau Patricia in Pacific Palisades (Kalifornien). Er ist Autor mehrerer geschichtlicher Werke und schreibt seit einigen Jahren an seiner Autobiographie "Mein Leben oder Der Ritt über den Bodensee".

## Über dieses Buch

Nach umfangreichem Studium des tragi-komischen Kampfes der "Overeater" ("Fresser") mit ihrer Gier vertritt Kellen in seinem kurzen Buch die radikale These, dass Fettleibigkeit nichts mit dieser oder jener Nahrungsaufnahme zu tun hat, sondern einzig und allein das Resultat einer psychologischen Eigenschaft ist – einer "blinden Dauergier", die man auflösen kann, wenn man sie als solche verstehen lernt. Kellens These: Diese "Dauergier" – und nicht Kalorien ganz gleich welcher Art – ist des "Fressers" Feind, den es für immer zu besiegen gilt. Jede Diät ist eine ungeeignete Waffe dafür.

# ABOUT THE AUTHOR

Konrad Kellen was a specialist in psychological operations with the U.S. Army in World War II. For his successful efforts he received the Legion of Merit. After the war, Kellen helped shape worldwide psychological operations for the U.S. Government in various government affiliated organizations. He retired from the Rand Corporation in Santa Monica, CA after 23 years as a senior staff member.

Konrad Kellen is the author of four books: *Khrushchev – A Political Portrait* (Fred A. Praeger Inc., 1961; *The French and Indian War* (Walker & Co., 1961); *The Coming Age of Woman Power* (Peter Wyden, Inc., 1972; *The Fall of South Vietnam* (Crane Russek, 1980).

Konrad Kellen has been a regular contributor to *MIDSTREAM Magazine* and *The New Leader.* He has written articles for *The New York Times Magazine, Los Angeles Times* "Opinion" section, *Esquire* magazine and others. His article on space exploration was reprinted in the Congressional Record. His article on GLUTTONY appeared in the October 1965 issue of the magazine *Mademoiselle* and was widely reprinted.

Konrad Kellen lives in Pacific Palisades, California. He likes to eat – and eat well.

## Über den Verleger und Herausgeber Dr. phil. Bernd A. Weil
(Selters-Eisenbach/Ts.)

geboren am 28. November 1953; Abitur; Studium der Germanistik, Politikwissenschaft, Geschichte und Diplom-Pädagogik in Frankfurt am Main; Verlagstätigkeit; Oberstudienrat, Diplom-Psychologe, Sozialpädagoge, Publizist und Verleger; Gutachter des Hessischen Kultusministers in Wiesbaden und verschiedener Institute; Rezensent der Bundeszentrale für politische Bildung in Bonn und der Gesellschaft für deutsche Sprache in Wiesbaden; zahlreiche Buchveröffentlichungen; Internet: www.bweil.de

## BUCHVERÖFFENTLICHUNGEN VON DR. BERND A. WEIL

1. SCHACH DEM TEUFEL. Erzählung in Anlehnung an die "Schachnovelle" von Stefan Zweig. Frankfurt/Main 1995 (ISBN 3-89501-221-1); DM 19,80

2. DER DEUTSCHE MINNESANG. Entstehung und Begriffsdeutung. Frankfurt/Main 1993 (ISBN 3-89406-783-7); DM 16,80

3. DIE SCHWARZSEHER. Satire. In: Frieling, Wilhelm Ruprecht (Hrsg.): Anthologie Buchwelt '94, Berlin 1993 (ISBN 3-89009-547-X); DM 29,80

4. NONSENS UND VERMISCHTES. Gedichte. In: Frieling, Wilhelm Ruprecht (Hrsg.): Anthologie Buchwelt '92, Berlin 1991 (ISBN 3-89009-270-5); DM 29,80

5. DIE REZEPTION DES MINNESANGS IN DEUTSCHLAND SEIT DEM 15. JAHRHUN-DERT, Frankfurt/Main 1991 (ISBN 3-89406-181-2); DM 68,--

6. DAS FALKENLIED DES KÜRENBERGERS. Interpretationsmethoden am Beispiel eines mittelhochdeutschen Textes. Frankfurt/Main 1985 (ISBN 3-88323-565-2); DM 9,80

7. GENERAL DR. VON STAAT. Zum Verhältnis von Militär und Politik zwischen 1919 und 1945. Frankfurt/Main 1985 (ISBN 3-88323-536-9); DM 18,--

8. FASCHISMUSTHEORIEN. Eine vergleichende Übersicht mit Bibliographie. Frankfurt/Main 1984 (ISBN 3-88323-528-8); DM 9,80

9. HEIMATBUCH: 750 JAHRE EISENBACH, GEMEINDE SELTERS (TAUNUS) (1234 bis 1984), Meinerzhagen 1984 (ISBN 3-88913-074-7)

10. KLAUS MANN: LEBEN UND LITERARISCHES WERK IM EXIL, Frankfurt/Main 1983 (ISBN 3-88323-474-5); DM 16,80

11. FABELN: VERSTEHEN UND GESTALTEN. Eine Unterrichtseinheit für die 8. Jahrgangsstufe. Frankfurt/Main 1982 (ISBN 3-88323-379-X); DM 16,80

# TABLE OF CONTENTS

# I.

# THE NATURE OF THE BEAST

# I. THE NATURE OF THE BEAST

To understand overeating, we must understand first, that while it is an addiction, it is not just another addiction like drugs, alcohol, or smoking. It is more insidious and therefore harder to overcome.

The drug addict, the alcoholic, the smoker can practice complete abstinence ("cold turkey"). Even then, the addiction remains beneath the surface, but it has become dormant and will be less nagging as time goes by.

The overeater does not have this "cold turkey" option. He must eat to stay alive. He is thus forever restimulating his appetite for food. The drug addict, the alcoholic, the smoker, can eventually "forget" the substance he craves. His body will "forget" it as well, at least to the point where it no longer nags at him. But the overeater is condemned to keep eating, to think about food, to decide when and where and what and with whom to eat. Therefore, if he wants to attain and maintain a desired weight, he must go through a more profound transformation than the drug or alcoholic addict. Can anyone see an alcoholic overcome his affliction if he had to forever take a few drinks three times a day in order to survive and function?

There is another reason why overeating is such an insidious and malignant habit: any single indulgence has no immediate discernible effects. If the abstaining alcoholic falls off the wagon just once, he is likely to get drunk, do things he later regrets, and suffers a hangover. But one more helping or one more piece of pie seems to make no different to anybody. It has no immediate effects. It does not slur the speech or cloud the mind. It does not lead to a traffic accident or tears by a spouse. The piece of pie seems innocuous and insignificant. And it is.

What is neither innocuous nor insignificant is the overeater's <u>response</u> to that piece of of pie. His morbid craving for it. His lost battle with it. That piece of pie is not the overeater's enemy. His enemy is his craving for it. His <u>gluttony,</u> not food, is his enemy. Gluttony is his overt and covert enemy, always lying in wait for him, even if he loses weight and keeps it off for a short while. For life without overeating seems not worth living for the glutton, even if he has the will power to intermittently stay slim. But will power is not what is needed to help the glutton reform. He must <u>dissolve</u> his gluttony. How to do that is the subject of this book.

To this (happy) end the glutton must first recognize what gluttony is. It is not a single trait or a bad habit. It cuts through his entire personality. And, like food or overweight, gluttony cannot be overcome by will power. For it is a <u>lack</u> rather than a _trait_. A lack cannot be torn out like a weed. It has to be filled with something else. What makes gluttony so powerful yet elusive is that it is a void, a yawning abyss. What the overeater feels so painfully is an emptiness, which he tries to fill with food. But this feeling of emptiness is not due to lack of food and cannot be sated with food. It is what causes his gluttony, which in turn is the result of many other obscure deficiencies and needs.

One should therefore think that psychiatry can cure the glutton of his addiction. But even the most ardent advocates and skilled practitioners of psychiatry admit that as a weapon against _any_ addiction their craft is powerless. Addictions can only be overcome by the victims, and then only if they first understand the roots of their addiction and the steps needed to curb it.

How long will that take? Only a fool would try to build a house in a day, and only a fool would hope to lose weight as quickly or easily as the diet books, diet pills, and diet clinics promise. To lose weight is not like tearing down a house, which can be done in a day. Rather, it is like building a house or a new person – a non-glutton – from the ground up.

Nothing can be fixed that is not understood and an end to overeating cannot be attained unless nature and causes and severity of the affliction of overeating are understood and accepted.    That takes time and patience, and neither is a glutton's strong suit,  but will also be very rewarding.    Like a child, he wants everything immediately, unconditionally and in infinite measure. That trait  — he will see upon sober reflection — is not conducive to shedding an ingrained vice and waltzing away a new person just by a "resolution." Impatience is the glutton's worst enemy: It makes him overeat; it makes him forever try spurious "quick weight loss" diets; it nails him ever more firmly to the cross of his gluttony. Like gluttony itself, his impatience with everything in life, including his gluttony, is his enemy.

## II. WHY LOSE WEIGHT?

Gluttony being a vicious circle, one can begin looking at it at any point. To ask <u>why</u> so many people are eager to lose weight is as good a starting point as any.

Three reasons are often given for the need or desire to lose weight:

- Weight loss makes a person healthier.
- It makes a person feel better.
- It makes a person more attractive.

And weight loss generally does lead to some attainment along these three goals. As they are clearly important goals, why are they not powerful enough to induce overeaters to mend their ways?

Reason (which is needed to produce <u>reasons</u>), as people have always suspected and as was demonstrated by Sigmund Freud, is not man's most powerful motivator, much as he wishes it were or tries to convince himself that it really is. Man wants to think of himself as "rational" and of his life style and his decisions as such also. But, alas, the evidence is that much of the time he and his decisions are not rational, and more unfortunately still, he often is not rational with regard to the most important matters in his life.

When a battle ensues between our reason, which weighs factors and reaches logical conclusions, and our unconscious, which makes blind and urgent demands, reason is often the loser. Not always, of course. Reason is not the loser when the equation of reason and impulse is more favorable to reason. This may occur when reason is very strong and impulse not so overpowering or enduring. But reason can be overcome by impulse in one fell swoop; it also can be eroded by Id's unrelenting pressure. This shows us that there are two kinds of overeating: "Impulse" overeating and "chronic" overeating. Of course, the two can overlap or even be indistinguishable.

But even the three reasons most frequently given for wanting to lose weight are not all grounded on a rational basis which  –  see above  –  is itself a feeble fundament. True, good or better health has a solid and rational appeal. But the prospect that the weight loser will feel better is uncertain. One can feel terrible even when one is healthy and of normal weight. Besides, feeling is subjective.

Apparently, the strongest yet most problematic desire for losing weight is the hoped for correlation between weight loss and attractiveness. One must suspect that the principal reason why most people want to lose weight is: <u>They want to look more attractive.</u> And they think that <u>looking</u> more attractive is <u>being</u> more attractive.

The first two reasons (better health and feeling better) are oriented toward oneself, the third (greater attractiveness) is connected with a person's social situation, his relations with others. Is it vanity? Unfortunately, vanity is a poor and unreliable motivator for any sustained or effective effort. Many people would like to be doctors or lawyers or movie stars out of vanity, to impress others. But the effort required to attain such roles in life, even if the necessary talents are present, require much more powerful motives than vanity. Vanity, like gluttony, is itself a void, a deficiency, an insatiable emptiness. Even if one can fight fire with fire, one cannot fight one deficiency with another.

Efforts at reducing based on vanity are rarely successful. In the rare cases where they do succeed, they produce a life hardly less tortured than it was when the overeater overate, since the craving for food is still with him; his efforts to lose weight are brutal, and his new figure does not bewitch all onlookers. Vanity and gluttony almost always go together. Of course, not every vain person is an overeater, but every overeater is likely to be a vain person. In this connection, "vain" not only means haughty and desirous of admiration, but also futile and empty. Vanity is futility and emptiness.

Efforts to lose weight based on vanity are, literally, vain. The feelings of human emptiness or lack, caused by vanity and the feelings of physical emptiness caused by gluttony converge and reinforce each other. Instead of trying to fight gluttony with vanity, the overeater would do better to fight both of them simultaneously.

There are several impulses related to vanity that tempt overeaters to reform. One is a form of hostility or disdain for "normal" people. Another is ambition, striving for superiority. There is also the desire to display one's triumph over one's peers. The overeater often feels hostility against his fellows who, like himself, hopelessly and eternally struggle against their vice. He is contemptuous of them, much as he is contemptuous of himself. He dreams of walking among them a different, slender person. He imagines himself proudly eating "everything" before their eyes without being an ounce overweight. He fantasizes about their amazement, admiration and envy.

There is much reason why the overeater wants to be envied. Overeaters usually are envious themselves, more than most people. The glutton is greedy, and the greedy person who always wants more than he can have is envious of others who seem to have what he lacks. In the case of a glutton, it is slimness and the ability to eat without retribution that is the target of his envy. But the desire to be envied fails to be a suitable or sufficient motivator to cut down our food because, like vanity, envy is a negative emotion. As already noted, one can't fight one deficiency with another.

The overweight person envies the person of normal weight because supposedly the latter is healthier, feels better, and is more attractive. But the real reason why overeaters want to be thin is that <u>they will then be able to eat all they want.</u> The overeater envies the slim person because he seems to be able to eat all he wants without getting fat. And this is true. A slim person eats all he wants, <u>not because he wants to be slim</u>, but because he doesn't <u>want</u> to eat more. If he wants more than he needs, his self-control is automatic and reliable.

But do not ordinary people also crave food? The answer is two-fold. They do get hungry and their hunger, if denied, can become very powerful. But that is not like the craving of the glutton, as the ordinary person's hunger is easily appeased. The ordinary person may also crave occasionally a certain food, but his craving will be different from the glutton's. *Playboy's* Hugh Hefner – clearly a thin person – while on a trip to Europe became, in his own words, "so horny for some home fried chicken" that he had some especially prepared for himself at Maxim's in Paris. Slim people, too, can experience a wild craving for "Mother's cooking," or for a big steak when they cannot find it. But such craving is selective and occasional. More significantly, it is satisfied when the craved food is consumed. The glutton's craving is never satisfied.

That continuous gorging and continuous slimness should coexist in the same person is the glutton's deepest wish. He wants to be thin in order to be able to eat more. And this is exactly what he does once he has "successfully" dieted. The first thing he will do when the scales finally show improvement is to eat more, with the inevitable result that no matter what his diet was, and no matter with how much pain it was observed, it is always undone again. For the glutton will do anything in the world, even diet, to eat more.

Most popular diets are advertised as having two aspects. One is that they allow the dieter to lose weight without suffering "hunger pangs;" the other is that "pounds will melt away." They thereby appeals to the glutton's passivity — they suggest he need not even make any active effort. Thus the implied purpose of most diets really is not the weight loss which can obviously be obtained simply by eating less without a particular plan, but to be a <u>palliative</u> to the glutton who wants to become slim but only if the road there is painless, i.e., if he can change his spots while remaining a tiger.

Why diet at all, if it is so unlikely to have a lasting effect? In fact, there really is no good reason to diet. It helps to eat less, but that is something else. Those who habitually do not eat more than they need are not gluttons and do not diet or otherwise restrict their eating. Only gluttons go on a diet. Non-gluttons do not crave more food than they need and therefore do not eat more than they need. They never go on diets. But the glutton, no matter how much or how little he eats, will always crave more food than he needs. He will therefore always be unhappy because he always will be either fat or hungry. Or, worse yet, both at the same time. Craving food and a slim body at the same time, he has a guarantee that he can never be satisfied no matter what he does.

This proves that systematically dieting or simply <u>trying</u> to eat less is not the answer. Nothing can be more futile than the glutton, on occasion, exchanging a rich appetizer with a chaste stick of celery. And he knows it. What he must do is surrender his gluttony. To this end he must change his personality so that his gluttony first abates and then dissolves. His dream should not be that his pounds melt away but that his gluttony melt away.

# III.  HAVING ONE'S CAKE

The overeater, to turn into a person of normal appetite and weight, must surrender his gluttony.  But, curiously, even though at times he may curse his craving for food, he is, without realizing it, attached to this craving.  He may <u>think</u> he would gladly surrender it if he could, but that is because he has not confronted or understood how attached to his appetite he really is.  Why is he so attached to something that torments him, that inflicts such cruel defeats on him, that makes him do things that are so damaging to himself?

The glutton loves his gluttony because without it he would not be able to experience his supreme and often only pleasure: to eat much and well.  The glutton has a different relationship to food than the non-glutton.  He may envy the non-glutton his effortlessly limited eating and slimness.  <u>But he definitely does not envy him his largely indifferent feeling about food.</u>  A non-glutton feels only mild pleasure or even indifference towards food while a glutton thrives on his ability to anticipate and savor "good" food.  He glows at the prospect.  His gluttony is a curse, on the one hand.  But it is also the capacity to derive intense delight and excitement out of something that others find only reasonably pleasurable, if at all.

The glutton who may curse his own "appetite" (i.e., his greed) would never want to change places with the kind of person who is indifferent to food. The glutton loves his sharp appetite for a good meal!

The glutton's gluttony is a powerful weapon with which he can temporarily defend himself against the miseries of the world. Give the glutton some bad news, let him suffer some loss or an indignity, and he will console himself with extra helpings. The non-glutton would lose his appetite in the same situation. Like the gambler or the alcoholic, the glutton can use his affliction — at least temporarily — as an anesthetic against all pain or boredom. A table laden with his favorite foods will take his mind off anything that troubles or pains him, including his gluttony.

When a glutton is on a diet or trying in some way to control his appetite, he will honestly deplore his affliction. But if you were to offer him a magic injection that would make him not crave food again — and thus deprive him of the exquisite expectation and satisfaction of mollifying his craving — he would refuse.

Like the person in the grip of an unhappy love affair, the glutton only wants satisfaction, not release. The unhappy lover, if offered a magic potion that would make him indifferent to his beloved, would also refuse, no matter how hopeless his situation or grievous his pain. The same goes for the glutton.

An overeater or over<u>craver</u> is a mass of contradictions. He does not want to be free of his desires, he wants to satisfy them. But he wants to satisfy them without gaining weight. He wants to eat and be slim at the same time. He wants to be able to get his euphoric pleasure out of food and not crave food at the same time. And if he can't have this, he eats to console himself.

Our contemporary unfortunate habit to equate all addictions with diseases can only accelerate the spread of <u>all</u> addictions. For a disease is something which the sufferer wants to get rid of as quickly as possible. There is no ambivalent attitude there. If certain hard steps are needed to heal pneumonia or a broken leg, the patient will gladly take them. But the addict loves one half of his vice. This is why he has such a hard time shedding it. And this is why it is so hard, if not impossible, for others to help him. For the sick person will generally be able and willing to do what is necessary. He will follow instructions without resisting because he wants to get well. But the addict will not and cannot do that.

If a person has a heavy cold and runs a high fever, it is easy for us to tell him he should take to his bed and do this or that. And it is easy for him to do it. But if a person is an alcoholic and we were to tell him, "Hey, you shouldn't drink!", he could and would not comply. So it is with the glutton. On the surface, his problem seems ever so simple: He should forever eat less. But he cannot and will not do this. His addiction may be a mental illness but it certainly is not an ordinary illness. Nor is alcoholism an illness any more than drug addiction or gluttony. Only our super-materialist "philosophy" can spread such nonsense.

Gluttony is evidence of what Freud called a character neurosis. It is a disturbance of the entire person, but usually short of incapacitating mental illness. This is proven by the fact that a simple head-on, direct assault on overeating never works, no matter what the advertised diet. In fact, dieting is without question a contributing cause of gluttony.

The reason is that any diet rivets the mind on food. This, for the glutton, is fatal. For, as a reluctant lover not only of food but of his gluttony as well, he tends to think more of food than ordinary people to begin with. And a diet makes him constantly think, calculate and calibrate food. And thinking about food and as a result craving it even more are one and the same thing for him.

But the glutton cannot stop eating because, no matter how reluctantly, he is attached to his gluttony which, when indulged, provides such deep pleasures. That does not mean he can simply stop loving his lust for food any more than a desperate but spurned lover can stop loving his beloved. He only can make his gluttony abate and disappear if he first understands it fully, which this small book will try to help him to do.

## IV.  THE IMPATIENT GLUTTON


Impatience is the reason we were driven out of Paradise.
And impatience is the reason we cannot reenter it.


Franz Kafka


Impatience is generally not attributed much importance in human affairs.  People may become irritated at times with the impatience of others, or try to curb their own on rare occasions.  But by and large they pay little attention to it.  Only rarely do they warn their children against it.  Essayists and psychologists do not write about impatience, novels rarely deal with it, poems have little to say about it.  One might say that people treat the subject of impatience itself with impatience, paying it scant attention, regarding it as a mere nuisance, if that.


But Kafka put impatience into the very center of the human experience.  Though he — a Western person — is unusual in this regard, he was not the only observer to do so.  Almost every Western person knows the oriental saying:  "Good things come to those who wait."  But Westerners pay little attention to that and regard it as irrelevant for their own lives.  They feel they cannot wait in our fast-moving world and fast-moving times.  They do not like to wait, or want to wait, or are able to wait.

One reason for this is that they do not distinguish between active and passive waiting. True patience is not just sitting there and waiting for something to happen. Rather, patience is the quality of giving things one does or wants to do, or that others do, the proper time to ripen.

To be patient about things in which we are not personally involved is easy. If we see a stranger who is grossly overweight we would say he might have a chance to reach a normal weight in, say, a year. If we then were to hear this person moan: "A year! Impossible! I must get rid of this fat in a few weeks," we would consider him not to be serious about his affliction.

But when it comes to ourselves it is a different matter. We don't easily assign the required time to our own efforts. And we avoid sustained efforts. Naturally, not all sustained effort is evidence of patience. A spurned lover who pursues the object of his desires for seven years may appear patient to us, but may not be that at all. He may be half crazed with impatience during the entire period. So it is with the glutton. He may have been dieting, off and on, for 20 years, which would make him appear as a paragon of patience to the naive observer. But, of course, he is not patient at all.

The glutton is more impatient than most people. His impatience focuses most strongly on the weight loss of which he dreams. But if he tries to take an indirect route toward reducing his craving for food (such as going to the movies, carrying on a conversation, or reading a book), his impatience is only temporarily "parked" in these substitute pursuits and flares up when they cease.

Psychiatry has an explanation for this. It declares the impatient person an oral personality, stuck in his emotional development at the level of a voracious infant. They attribute to him the need or desire to have anything he wants (as already stated above) "immediately, unconditionally, and in infinite measure." The psychiatrists are probably right, as far as it goes. But the glutton is not served with this description of himself, whether he consciously accepts or rejects it.

Fortunately, there are other ways to look at the roots of a glutton's impatience. We are talking here about morbid, basic, chronic impatience, not the impatience of a person stuck with a defective car on the way to the airport. The impatience of which we speak is tied in with a faulty perception of time: what time is, what it does, how it flows. The impatient person wishes that what he wants to do should take less time than it actually does or that he would like to devote to it. In fact, he wishes things would not "take" any time at all. He wants things immediately.

That is why successful but phony diet merchants always advertise their promise of weight loss as "fast" and "immediate." That is how they land their fish, who would not go for the promised weight loss if it were not "fast." Just as the glutton is a sitting duck for the word "effortless," he is a sitting duck for the word "fast." He may be brilliant in other ways, but the word "fast" has such a hypnotic effect on him that it blots out all his reasoning powers.

That is not only because the glutton craves weight loss as avidly as he craves food, but because his relationship to time is seriously deranged. He always feels his time is very limited, be it the time to get all the things he thinks he needs, be it the time left to accomplish or enjoy things, be it his time on earth. Related to this is his feeling that he is already way behind; that for a variety of reasons, including his gluttony, he has gotten fewer of those desirables (success, love, admiration, security) than others or than he should have gotten.

He sees life as a race in which he is always several laps behind and the prize money is always going to those ahead of him.

And so his impatience increases.

Time is so precious to a glutton that he will not voluntarily "take" enough of it for anything. And so he *nolens volens* keeps wasting it in large measure. He wastes it by doing the same thing over and over that has already failed. His problem is that he has not developed a normal relationship to time.

Let us engage in a simple exercise. Suppose a glutton were told on the sixth of June of a specific year that as of tomorrow morning – the seventh of June – his weight will be exactly normal. Within the next 24 hours he will have shed all excess weight. Would that be soon enough for him? It would indeed. He would be euphoric at the prospect.

If then we were to ask him: "But isn't that too late?" He would consider that a dumb question. Certainly not, he would say.

Yet, had we asked him one or two or ten years earlier whether that particular day, the seventh of June of that year, would be an acceptable target date for him to be of normal weight, he wouldn't have consented. He would have said: "What? A year, or two, or ten? My dear fellow, I haven't got that kind of time."

And thus the one or two or ten years passed, whether he felt he could let them pass or not. And he is still overweight.

Then, like the gambler who always increases his stakes when he is losing (for he, too, is heedlessly impatient), the glutton sets for himself ever more stringent time limits, because he has "lost" so much time already, and therefore has so little time left to (1) become slim, and (2) harvest, belatedly, all the delights slimness will bring.

The glutton lives in the past on the one hand, and in the future on the other, disregarding (and wasting) the present. And because of his impatience, time that is really short seems long to him. What is a year? A long or a short time? That depends on what it is used for or what we expect we can accomplish in the course of it. If, in a year or even two, we could attain a normal weight and the frame of mind needed to maintain it by alleviating or extinguishing our gluttony, would that not be a very short time, considering that we may have worked on our weight and food consumption for 20 or more heartrending years? It would be a short time indeed in retrospect, but the glutton cannot see this in prospective in his blind impatience. He will impatiently dismiss any person who would tell him how he could normalize and stabilize his weight in a year or two. It doesn't interest him in the least.

Tied in closely with impatience is procrastination. The glutton is one of the world's worst procrastinators. In this he is not alone — it is a common disease today. Overwhelmed by the endless work of modern life, people postpone whatever they think they can get away with postponing.

But procrastination is the thief of time. It can also be very painful. It poisons the time the procrastinator gains by postponing his tasks. Being always far behind, he always feels guilty. Thus he fails to enjoy the time "for himself" he thinks he can "carve out" by postponing things.

The fact that procrastination is so widespread in our time makes it no less serious. Sometimes it is tempting to regard something as harmless just because it is so widespread, but that is foolish and often dangerous. The Black Death in the 13<sup>th</sup> century was so widespread that almost half the people fell victim to it, yet it could not be regarded as harmless merely because it was so common. Both procrastination and gluttony are extremely common. Consequently, those in their grip mistakenly tend to dismiss them as of little consequence.

The procrastinator behaves like a person who has all the time in the world. He always seems to be thinking about new efforts. He talks about them endlessly. Sometimes he will even go so far as to undertake some. But he never follows through to the finish. It is as if it made no difference whether he "gets around to it" tomorrow, the next week, or the next year.

In the same way, the glutton always talks and thinks about losing weight. But then he postpones the diet. Or he goes off it, in order to get back onto it after some more time has elapsed.

In addition, he invariably finds that external circumstances seem to conspire endlessly and mysteriously in favor of his interrupting or postponing a better eating regime. As soon as he has grimly determined to abstain from everything not sanctioned by the great doctors Mayo, Pritikin, Tarnower, or Stillman, an avalanche of dinner invitations comes crashing into his house. Or Aunt Henrietta, 80 years old and nearly blind, has baked a rich cake for his birthday and wants to see him taste an extra large slice. How can he refuse? It is as though the gods are mocking him, forcing him forever to postpone his "diet."

But other things, too, force him to postpone his diet (or break it, i.e., postpone it until "later"). His boss has scowled at him. His beloved seems to have been a trifle cold during the last amorous encounter. His son has fallen off his bike. His insurance premium has doubled. All this calls for consolation  –  food. Conversely, good things may have happened: He received a promotion. One of his enemies has bitten the dust. An effort of his triumphed. The annual physical checkup has not confirmed some dire suspicions. Such things will then have to be celebrated. With food, of course. In the life of a glutton, _everything_ that happens calls for a copious meal, either for the purposes of celebration or consolation.

In the overeater, the desire for more food than is needed is an automatic response, a reflex, a constant trigger that is pulled by everything, including a hated weight gain. Nor does this only apply to the present. The glutton's appetite may be intolerably triggered by the mere thought of an indignity he suffered 20 years ago, or by a foolishness he committed last night. But contrary to other reflexes, such as laughing, sneezing, or shrinking from an expected blow, which are triggered only by special stimuli, the glutton's appetite is triggered by everything. Therefore, there is no escape in procrastination, as there are always new reasons to postpone a change in eating habits.

The procrastinator's lot is an unhappy and frustrating one. He does not postpone things because he has the time to do so, but because he has so many seemingly compelling reasons to do so. As he is also a very impatient person, this postponement, though brought on by himself, can be very painful. His anxiety, which is already at a high level because he thinks he has so little time left for anything, increases with every postponement. Even more time will now be needed than was originally planned.

Craving time and quick results (in the same way that he craves good), yet suffering interminable delays due to continuous postponements, the overeater is confronted and plagued by the same contradictions he suffers in other fields. Concerning food reduction he behaves, simultaneously, as though he had very little time and all the time in the world. He would never accept a regime that would promise him normal weight and eating habits in two year, but he will diet for 20! Plagued by this hopelessly contradictory perception and use of time, the glutton will want to turn his mind from the problem. He has no alternative but . . . to eat.

It always helps understanding to look at the origin of words. The word im-patience means an inability or unwillingness to suffer -- suffer whatever needs to be suffered (patience and pathology deriving from the Greek root "path," to suffer). There are many reasons why the glutton is so unwilling to suffer, not the least of which is that he is a chronic sufferer to begin with, unable or unwilling to shoulder any suffering additional to what he already and habitually carries.

## V.  TO EAT LIKE A PIG


If you want to stop drinking,

watch a drunk while you are sober.


Chinese Proverb


We live in an age in which we pride ourselves on being rational enough to solve most problems with our analytical ability, and social enough to be dispassionate: to understand everything and condemn nothing. *Tout comprendre c'est tout pardonner* is, unfortunately, a widely accepted posture. This type of pseudo-generous thinking has stunted and even destroyed millions of lives.


If we look, say, at a criminal who has done great harm to some of his fellow creatures, it is worthwhile to try to understand what turned him into such a person. And, in some way, we might then even forgive him. But that does not mean that we should declare him innocent or regard him as sick or disturbed and try to rehabilitate him (he was not "habilitated" to begin with, so how can he be "rehabilitated"?) with the help of social workers who may be as much in need of habilitation as he is.

The dubious concept of total understanding leading to total forgiveness has been carried over into the fields of alcohol and drug addiction, much to the detriment of those afflicted. We live in an age not only of obstinate permissiveness, but in the age of <u>tutelage</u>. We recommend treatment for the criminal as we do for the child abuser or any other kind of social derelict. We even decide that terrorist hostages held in captivity will require weeks of counseling before they can return to society. Are they infants?

Underlying all such concepts is that what used to be called crimes and what used to be called vices are now declared to be manifestations of illness. Criminals and addicts are regarded as victims of forces over which they have no control. It is, in other words, "not their fault." So if I have done or am doing bad things to myself or others because of forces over which I have no control, no one can blame or condemn me. That is, of course, very nice.

But there is another, sinister side to the same coin. If something I did was indeed caused by forces over which I had no control (which makes me a victim of sickness rather than a perpetrator of crime or the practitioner of a vice), then I'm condemned not ever to be able to change my behavior. How could I change it if it is conditioned by forces outside my control?

This contemporary view of man offers him all the freedom in the world to behave badly (the largest corporations in the country have now "recognized" alcoholism as an illness and have spent millions treating it); but it also deprives a person of the power to improve or change himself. In the contemporary view he is as nothing, just a helpless victim. Thus is he condemned to remain a drunk or drug addict or criminal forever? No, says that same society; he is sick; he can be cured.

What our society really does is to "spoil" such people in the way indiscriminately permissive parents spoil their children. A contemporary social observer or activist might refuse to condemn a slovenly and habitual drunk as worthless and contemptible. But the drunk knows he is worthless and contemptible, at least in his more lucid moments, just as the naughty child knows he is behaving poorly and deserving of some discipline.

If society expressed some measure of contempt and disapproval for people whose behavior is objectionable and damaging to themselves and others — as society has done for thousands of years before the invention of the social sciences — such people would at least have the advantage of being taken seriously, of being judged by normal standards. They would not be written off as incapable of change by their own efforts, of being victims rather than victimizers. Public contempt for certain behaviors and traits is not a medieval or benighted thing. On the contrary, it can be a powerful help for the members of that society to attain constructive and satisfying lives despite the temptation, present in most of us, to just let go, relinquish all efforts at being civilized, and sinking into sloth and vice.

Hard though it may seem to accept, and harsh, too, there is something contemptible about an overeater. "Modern" society will reject this as a shocking statement, but the glutton, who is that statement's actual target, is likely to accept it. He knows himself better than society knows him.

Most of us do react adversely when we see someone "making a pig of himself." We may detest or we may pity him. But we will certainly feel pity and even disdain if we know he is making a pig of himself habitually AGAINST HIS WILL.

Just as people in the Middle Ages did not consort with people whom they considered to be possessed by demons, we do not like to look at or associate with people who are in the grip of vices they try to but are powerless to control. That is, unless we are one of them. As we already said, this accounts for the camaraderie and good fellowship of thieves, sex offenders, drug addicts – and gluttons. It is not a true camaraderie, but rather a congregating of outcasts who feel less outcast, less guilty, less detestable when in the company of similar outcasts. In fact, with a psychological sleight of hand, <u>they</u> often detest society. Drunks and drug users tend to think and claim that others are squares and have no fun. Gluttons likewise tend to regard non-gluttons as unrefined and unhedonic. They pity those who cannot rave over a two-pound lobster.

But the reality is otherwise. The glutton who is powerless at the thought or sight of food, especially when his dearest wish in life is to be slimmer, is in fact not an admirable person. Of course, it is not the cake or gravy or French fries that are his undoing, but it is the underlying force, his gluttony, the emptiness within him and his ignorance of the mainsprings of his affliction. These diabolical forces are no laughing matter. The glutton remains, outwardly at least, the helpless victim of a salami sandwich or a second helping of ice cream, and we are inclined to look down on that.

Unfortunately for the glutton, society curbs its impulse of showing its disdain, granting him instead the absolution of a guiltlessly acquired neurosis which he cannot shed. The glutton would be better off if we expressed our true feelings, however. To be looked down on, to be regarded as ridiculous and as hopelessly handicapped and confused, and, if the glutton is a dieter, as being entangled in a hopeless fight against windmills, could be quite a curative shock. Too bad our society forbids its application. It leaves the glutton without social controls or support. Therefore he must <u>himself</u> face the fact that he "eats like a pig." That should be quite bracing for him in his battle to overcome his affliction.

We have said that the glutton is spoiled. The word has two meanings: to wreck or destroy or impair something, or to give a person something extra, something to which he is not entitled, something he should and need not have. In French, the word is exactly the same. *Gater* means to spoil, and *un enfant gâté* is a spoiled child. In German, the semantics are different. A spoiled child is a *verwoehntes Kind. Verwoehnt* is a word of different origin than "spoiled," but it is equally enlightening as to the nature of the affliction. Literally, *ver-woehnt* means mal-habituated, or "having been given bad habits." Does this not describe spoiled people, including gluttons, perfectly? Finally, in Spanish, a spoiled child is a *nino consentido*. This means a child that has been "consented to" too much, that learned to get away with what it should not have been gotten away with. Does not the glutton get a flash of self-recognition here?

## VI.  GAMES GLUTTONS PLAY

Like other people in the grip of their vices, gluttons are rarely straight with others or themselves. They are, especially, <u>fake</u> believers in <u>quick fixes</u>.

No diet is popular with them unless it promises <u>fast</u> weight loss. This is in line with the impatience we have mentioned, which is a trademark of every glutton and a sign of his infantile personality. Not only is he oral in his needs and impulses, but he craves immediate gratification, be it for food when he wants to eat, be it for weight loss when he wants to reduce, be it for applause if he loses a couple of pounds.

Every glutton knows in his heart that quick weight loss is impossible to attain, i.e., true weight loss. Yes, one can lose several pounds in a few days through water loss, but that is no true weight loss. Even a few pounds of actual fat can be shed rather quickly by some. But a quick loss of substantial weight cannot be attained even on a starvation diet. Every glutton, and especially every glutton who ever dieted, knows that. Yet he still insists on a quick weight loss diet. And he makes himself believe that it works if in a week or two he has lost a few pounds.

Beyond that, ever dieting glutton knows that even if he sticks to a diet he will not be able to keep his weight down. But he says and pretends he will. Of course, a diet is in itself a game, designed to fail, at least if it is a reducing diet. (There are other diets, such as salt-free diets for people with high blood pressure, or sugar-free diets for diabetics, which can be observed indefinitely and serve a good purpose.) But the purpose and target of any reducing diet is to <u>end it</u> sooner or later, at which point the old eating habits take over with doubled force. While the diet lasts, the weight loss, especially if it is relatively quick, brings about no basic changes, so that the body literally bounces back when once again fed as before.

Gluttons know this. But dieting itself is a part of the game they play, and a contributing cause to even greater gluttony. They scour the magazines in search of diets the way some people scour porno mags for ever-new photos. They search for new "painless" diets (especially new "miracle" diets) like astronomers search for new constellations. They do know that all these efforts are doomed, as the "miracle" diets are unobservable and provide at best non-lasting relief either from weight or from gluttony. The gluttons know, above all, that a diet that allows them to shed weight without his suffering "hunger pangs" does not and cannot exist. But they keep looking for and reading and talking about it.

Why does such a "miracle" diet not exist? One reason is that most people do not suffer less hunger pangs when they diet for a while. The less most people eat, the less they want food, as long as they get enough food to stay alive. But the glutton's greed is not for nourishment; it is for the pleasure involved in feasting his eyes, his nose and his palate, and for the feeling of being full, of having filled the yawning void. These cravings remain, no matter what the diet that is being tried. They are the result of a character disorder that the glutton, if he truly wants to cease being one, must face.

Therefore, as a beginning, he must stop playing games. This is a step he can take without much further understanding of what really ails him. Even if he can't give up overeating for a long time to come, he can give up playing games with himself and others.

The first game he must surrender, no matter how addicted he may be to that, too, is dieting. He must throw out all his diet books and clippings, and he must stop reading about diets in his favorite magazines.

He must face the fact that he has more than a good problem, that he has a character disorder that makes him unhappy far beyond his eating and his weight, and that no diet can make a dent in that. Earlier we said that gluttony, not food, is the enemy of the overeater. We can add now that all diets are likewise his enemy, as they cannot and do not work. Worse, they are counterproductive, as they keep him riveted to a game in which he can only lose.

## VII.  THE GLUTTON AND HIS SCALES

Whereas people who have no weight problem hardly ever weigh themselves (and generally do not even know how much they weight), every glutton has scales and he constantly weighs himself and knows exactly what he weighs.  Doesn't that tell us something?

Here as elsewhere, reality is different from the glutton's dream or perception.  The glutton thinks: "If only I had that slim body of the fellow down the aisle, I would step on the scales three times a day and exult!"  He probably fancies that the slim fellow does exactly that.  Anyway, that's what he thinks he would do if he were that fellow.

But that fellow with the slim figure rarely, if ever, steps on the scales.  Even more incredibly for the glutton, he derives no particular pleasure from his normal weight.  Just as the non-glutton does not derive the mad delight from his food that the glutton does, the non-glutton does not derive mad pleasure from seeing the scales show his decent weight that the glutton would experience if he could ever reach that point.  The non-glutton simply is not all that morbidly interested in his weight, just as he is not all that interested in food.

Thus, since one way of becoming a non-glutton is to do as non-gluttons do, the glutton must not diet, nor must he weight himself regularly. He must understand that just as he is obsessionally interested in and concerned with food, so is he with his weight. This excessive interest is all part of the same package, of the same vicious circle. The glutton must try to break it wherever he can.

Why is the glutton so concerned with his weight? We have seen overweight people burst into tears when they gained two or three pounds, and exult when they lost the same amount. This seems almost insane to the non-glutton or ex-glutton. But there are several reasons for these exaggerated responses, all of them based on erroneous perceptions. The glutton who sees he has gained a few pounds is terror-stricken because he thinks that, at whatever point his weight is, he is once again irreversibly on the way up, just as he greatly overestimates the loss of a few pounds as indication that he is now on the way down, and that he thinks he has gained control over his affliction.

Especially, a glutton's excessive responses to relatively insignificant gains or losses of weight are tied in with his impatience and demand for quick effects. He never considers that if his gluttony were made to dissolve he would weigh 20 or 30 pounds less in a year or two, regardless of small fluctuations; and that, unless he loses his gluttony, small fluctuations are irrelevant, be they up or down.

The glutton sees his scales as an instrument of either castigation or reward. If he has been "good" the scales will reward him, if he was "bad" they will punish him. And as the scales are more likely to punish than reward him, they are a holy terror in his bathroom.

Throw them out! Live like a non-glutton who may have them but rarely uses them. At least it would be a beginning. If the emulation of a role model helps drug addicts or alcoholics (and it does) to free themselves from their curse, why should gluttons not take non-gluttons as role models and try to emulate them and their ways? They will not be able — at least in the beginning — to assume the same stance toward food as the non-glutton, or eat sensibly. But they can imitate non-gluttons by stopping dieting or weighing themselves constantly. They will at first find it extremely hard not to weigh themselves, especially in case of weight loss which they are so excessively eager to see registered on the scales. However, to try will be good exercise.

The glutton's excessive concern with his weight, like with his diet or his food, only exacerbates his affliction. It can be curbed only if it is understood. This excessive concern with his weight is an excessive concern with his figure and appearance and thus, ultimately, with himself. It is evidence of this narcissism, just as his gluttony is, just as his dream of losing weight and then impressing and bewitching others is. The glutton, if he wants to cease being one, must learn to get off himself. This includes

getting off his scales.

# VIII.  TALKING ABOUT FOOD

Constant and emphatic talk about food is the unmistakable hallmark of the glutton. When the glutton does not eat, he talks about food, and when he does not talk about food, he thinks about it.

The uninitiated may think these are harmless pleasures. They are not. They can be traced directly to the overeating that results. What counts here is that the glutton's excessive (perpetual) interest in food drives out other interests. Or it may be the result or lack of other interests to begin with. This is one thing that is at the core of the glutton's affliction and character disorder: an insufficient interest in the world at large, in matters other than food, in other activities and other enjoyments.

As cause or as a result, the glutton's mind is riveted on food. He thereby thinks and talks up a storm of an appetite in himself. When we say here that talk about food is the glutton's enemy, we mean this in the broadest sense including the written word about food. Just as people morbidly interested in sex, when reading a book, come to full attention only when there are sex scenes, the glutton reads voraciously (quite literally) when in fact or fiction big and exquisite meals are described.

But just as he <u>can</u> throw away his scales, the glutton can stop talking about food or listening to others who do. Like the discarding of his scales and his diets, he will find this helpful in leading his mind first away from food, and then into other channels. In fact he will find it a relief! This should set a beneficial circle into effect, in that when the mind works in other channels, thoughts about food will be further curbed.

To the non-glutton, it is incredible how central a glutton's thought and preoccupation with food really is. When the glutton goes to a meeting or on a business trip, his first thoughts are of the food he will be served. When a friend just returned from Paris or Africa, his first questions will be what the friend ate there. As said before, this is not simply evidence of the glutton's affliction, it also adds to the affliction by stimulating it further.

Now, whereas the glutton cannot control his eating, at least not in the beginning, he can to some extent control his thinking and talking about food. This is an excellent first exercise, suited to curb his obsession. It must begin with a glutton's self-examination of how much, and in what ways, he really thinks, talks, or reads about food when not actually eating.

In this connection, the glutton — like any other addict — always seeks out but is badly served by the company of fellow sufferers from the same affliction. A glutton's worst enemy is a fellow glutton who makes him overcome his guilt and talk more about food and then eat more. But gluttons congregate because misery likes company, and gluttony is misery (even if it does seem to be the opposite when we see a glutton's feast at a heavily-laden table).

The talk and thought about food is also a thought about oneself; and as the thought about himself is depressing for the glutton, and as depression (like all other emotions) stimulates his appetite, thought about himself (as distinguished from honest thought about his affliction) also seduces him to eat more. So close is food to the glutton's heart that any interest in food is well nigh an interest in his own heart, i.e., himself.

## IX.  FOOD AND SEX

Though many people suffer from some kind of sexual dysfunction who are neither drug addicts nor alcoholics or gluttons, there seem to be no alcoholics, drug addicts or gluttons who do not have their sexual troubles.  This is not necessarily a result and consequence of their addiction only.  They already had sexual troubles before they became addicted to food, liquor or drugs.  Among those to whom we talked, there was no glutton, male or female, who had a satisfactory love and sex life.  All had functional troubles in that area, and all craved more and better sex.

It seems that just as for gluttons food is a substitute, sex is also a substitute.  Therefore they perform sex poorly, or lack sex altogether.  And the negative image most gluttons have of their bodies aggravates the problem.

Somehow, the entire sensorium of a person demands gratification, and if that cannot be obtained, the person will do two things:  find a substitute gratification that is easily available, and deaden, at least to some extent, that demanding sensorium.  Food, like drugs or alcohol, provides substitute gratification for sex and also deadens the senses at the same time if real satisfaction is not possible.

For the average glutton this insight is of no immediate value. He can throw away his diet books or his scales, and he can curb his talk and even his thinking about food, but he cannot step out and provide a satisfactory sex life for himself all at the same time.

Yet, if he changes his ways as thoroughly as he will have to if he wants to liberate himself from his gluttony, a better sex life will result, which will then in turn further reduce what may be left of his gluttony. As distinguished from the vicious circles chaining the glutton to his cross of food, there are also beneficial circles for him if he can dissolve his vice.

A hint: Unsatisfactory sexuality seems often connected with excessive self-concern and narcissism. This leads to morbid shyness and poor performance. It therefore also leads to a dearth of partners, since narcissistic and shy people with excessive self-concern and limited interests tend to be not very exciting or attractive to others. Once gluttons manage to have wider interests, they will also have wider choices. But it takes much time and effort first to get off of oneself, at least to a reasonable degree.

Naturally, once a more satisfactory sex life is attained, interest in food that is of a compulsive and surrogate nature will automatically decline.

Unfortunately, this is a devilish subject. Just as food is often a substitute for other satisfactions, so is sex. The question therefore arises: Can one substitute be driven out or (satisfactorily) replaced or driven out by another substitute? The writer has an easy answer: He does not know.

## X. THE JOGGING GLUTTON

Some people jog because they like it. Others jog because they have been told it is good for their health. The glutton jogs because he wants to work off some of that extra food he was unable to deny himself and the extra weight he carries like a slave carries his burden. But he wants to work it off so that he can eat more the next time.

Though he is told on impeccable authority that he must run practically once around the earth to work off just one extra lamb chop, or play seven sets of tennis to neutralize a jelly donut, he loves to exercise and especially to jog.

Why?

One answer is simple. In jogging, a person sweats. And a person who sweats, though he loses little real weight, other than water weight, will see a lower figure on the scales immediately after he stops jogging.

So the glutton jogs primarily in order to be able to eat more with a better conscience. This means he now has two scourges instead of one — eating and jogging. Jogging can be a scourge indeed, physically, mentally and morally. Physically it is hard to do because for an adult it simply is not natural to run. Children always run and love to run. For adults it is an unsuited and unnatural method of locomotion. So unnatural is it, in fact, that we not only do not like to run ourselves but we do not even like to see other adults run. Especially overweight people! True, the sinewy, muscular young jock, when running or jogging, can look pretty good, in fact enviably so. But that is because he doesn't need to lose weight, he already has a perfect build which he moves vigorously and gracefully. For most of us, jogging is unnatural.

Mentally, jogging can also be very trying. It's boring for most people, even people who do not need constant diversion when alone or in company. While jogging, they can neither talk, not read, nor really think about anything. So, nowadays, many joggers wear headphones that pump noise or nonsense into their crania, which can drive anyone to overeating later!

Finally, morally, jogging is probably the greatest hazard. For the glutton, who is a notorious backslider when it comes to curbing his appetite, is more than likely a notorious backslider and procrastinator in the area of jogging as well. This will give him more of what he is eminently prone to already: a bad conscience. Now, when he overeats and fails to jog as much as he had planned to, his bad conscience will be fed from two sources instead of one. No easy fate.

In general, contrary to legend, exercise can do very little for the overeater, because so much exertion is needed to work off so little weight. This does not mean that exercise (other than jogging) is not good for the overeater, for other reasons, if he keeps it on a sensible level. Exercise will keep him fitter and healthier and also somewhat less unhappy. It will make him look more attractive which is one of his anxious concerns. It will keep him in better physical and mental shape all around. It may even help him indirectly with regard to his weight problem by affecting his eating habit, in that good exercise reduces the appetite and stimulates his mind, reducing his cravings. Nothing stimulates the overeater's hunger more than inaction. Actually, this is not all that surprising, in that inaction contributes heavily to frustration and impatience, which in turn are the mainsprings of the glutton's gluttonous appetite.

## XI.  BOREDOM

One of the glutton's worst enemies is his boredom. The boredom need not be constant, though in some of the more unfortunate of us it is. But even when dormant, it is ever-present in the glutton, ready to spring on its victim. This is why food is of such consuming (sorry!) interest to him. His interest in other things or people is so weak or fleeting that food exerts and imposes itself on him as the most interesting thing to think about and use. He is <u>obsessed</u> by food: Food literally sits on him, ruling and steering and oppressing him, like the monkey that it is, on his back. It is indeed his obsession. (The word derives from the Latin *sedere*, to sit, and *ob*, meaning on top.)

This brings us right back to the void, or emptiness, the glutton vainly tries to fill with food. It is an emptiness that is present all over, not just in his gut. His head feels empty too. The images of roast duck, poached salmon, and lemon meringue pie slip only too easily into that empty head, assuming a life of their own and nagging him to act on them and find and eat them all.

The overeater's lack of interest in people  —  except perhaps for one generally unattainable love object visualized or pursued as the ideal partner for romance  — leads the glutton to "love" food instead. The excessive demands of his palate are not

63

just substitutes for other sensory satisfactions for whose pursuit he has insufficient inclination or ability. They also are substitutes for the love he would lavish on other people (or receive from other people) if he had the emotional maturity for that. But he hasn't. In fact, so immature is he on the unconscious emotional level that the need to love and the need to devour are one, as they are, it seems, in infants.

What makes food so attractive in addition is that it is defenseless. One can devour it and it will not resist. The love of food can be indulged without the need for reciprocation from the object of one's love.

Due to his basic impatience and to his basic shyness, which he often mistakenly attributes to his overweight appearance, the glutton is not the world's best communicator. Moreover, he tends to be rigid and demanding. Generally, the number of his friends is small, and the number of those he loves and who love him even more so. He really does not care much about his fellow gluttons, as already said; he seeks their company (and they his) mainly for sharing the lust provided by food. But they don't really interest him.

These feelings of inadequacy in turn alienate other people. The glutton feels rejected and he resents it. Resentment, in turn, leads to passivity, which leads to boredom and inaction. Then the glutton eats more than other people <u>and</u> works off less of the food he consumes when "stewing in his own juice" and being bored. And boredom leads to resentment which breeds dullness and vice-versa. This shows that the glutton who resents a lot of things tends to be a dullard, a <u>bore</u>. This ties in with the single-mindedness of his pursuit of food and brings us to yet another peculiarity of the glutton which deepens his propensity to eat and also his misery: He not just talks about food, as said earlier, quoting flawlessly form the menus of famous restaurants, he also talks about food and his <u>diet</u>, which bores most non-gluttons.

Naturally, among overeaters, the talk is either on food or on diets. Diets the gluttons has read about, heard about, tried and tested, or expects to go on. When it comes to diets he has heard about, he will tell – and believe – stories that will outdo a Baron Muenchhausen. But they will not outdo his fellow gluttons. There is always a tale about this man or that woman who lost 10 pounds in the first 10 days and, mind you, without once going hungry! Fabulous!

For others and for himself, one of the worst traits of an overeater, as of an alcoholic, is that he always lets the whole world know that he is swearing off or has sworn off food. Then, when he falls off the wagon, food-wise, he has to stomach the humiliation of having to eat his words about his expected accomplishments which once again turned to ashes. Humiliation is something the glutton is very sensitive to and feels chronically in any event.

The glutton should consider that this is equally true for the smoker who generally announces with a hopeful grin that he has quit smoking only to have failed *coram publico* a short time later when we see him surreptitiously puffing away.

In any event, nothing is more boring than failed reducing efforts by the glutton and for the glutton.

## XII.  THE GLUTTON'S ASSETS

Is it possible that an overeater has followed this author through all these pages which have told him only negative and (he thinks) discouraging things about his gluttony? If that is the case, he will now hear things that may please him and give him comfort.

The glutton is and has always in his life been a sufferer. Suffering can purify and sensitize a person. It can make him, at least potentially, more aware, more responsive, more appreciative than others. Under no conceivable conditions did the overeater have a happy childhood. Although an unhappy childhood may breed all the bad qualities to which the human race is heir, and the glutton carries his share of them, it also often makes people keener to the plight of others, gives them a broader view and often even a sense of humor.

Quite often, the glutton is also more intelligent than other people, and also more talented. It is a curious and unjust feature of life that unusual gifts and capabilities often represent such a burden for the individual that he seeks to deaden rather than develop them. For talents, too, can be merciless and over-stimulating slave drivers. It is ironic that many talented and creative people are poor managers of their own selves and their own resources. In history, they often were alcoholics or slaves to other addictions. Their greater sensitivity that enables them to experience more things than others, and more profoundly at that, can be a heavy burden and a disruptive factor for them. This sensitivity can be a two-edged sword, in that it can imprison a person in his isolation and in his gluttony until he re-forms himself; but it also can actually help him to re-form and become more attuned to his surroundings.

The glutton's bad qualities are generally endured by him only reluctantly. He is at odds with himself, split in half in the most painful fashion, schizophrenic in a dozen ways — due to his ambivalent and contradictory nature.

The truly "bad boy" of whom there are so many in our society, from gas station robber to rapist, from burglar to murderer and white-collar criminal, embodies no such contradictions. He is a piece of a whole cloth. His bad qualities have no countervailing features, which is also why not one in a hundred is ever rehabilitated. In fact, most of these "bad boys" are proud of their bad qualities, regarding them as manly.

Not so the glutton. The glutton is different. <u>He is a bundle of emotional contradictions, and therein lies his hope.</u>

Also, just as the glutton is rarely altogether evil or a burden on society, he is rarely altogether crazy. True, he is prey of some severe illusions. But he is usually not psychotic. He is not a paranoid schizophrenic. Significantly, however different insane people may be from each other, they are almost always slim. And so, generally, are professional criminals. Not the glutton!

But the overeater has many good qualities in reserve which he can mobilize. And he has much hidden realism about himself which he can bring to bear on his affliction. Above all, he is a striver, albeit not a successful one — so far. But, as the German poet Goethe said: "Whoever keeps striving can find salvation." This pertains directly to the glutton. He can be saved, or, more precisely, he can save himself.

It may seem that the list of good qualities attributed here to the glutton is very short. True, but it is also very weighty.

## XIII.  WHAT MUST THE GLUTTON BECOME?

Even though our age is regarded by many as the age of analysis, most perplexed people do not much care what is happening, be it in Russia, in the United States, or in themselves. They merely want to know:  "What should I do?"

In the modern bureaucracy, thousands of pages of analysis on missile strategy, international detente, world hunger, rising crime, and other subjects are produced at the cost of billions of dollars. But nobody really reads them. The busy, high-powered players who have at least a modicum of power to alter conditions, only look for the barest summaries (General George Marshall never read a memo of more than one page). Mostly they seek only "recommendations" from an army of analysts which they then disregard.    And rightly so, for those recommendations are always a disappointment. It does not matter what they say  —  they are either impossible to implement, or they contain nothing new.

It is not that the academic analysts are all stupid.  Rather, it is that most of their thinking on multifaceted, complicated, and fundamental questions is simplistic. Crime, hunger, national security have no solutions. The only thing a person concerned with them can do is engross himself into the realities of the situation, listen to open-ended views of other observers, and hope to stimulate other minds to have new insights leading to more realistic action.

For the glutton, his gluttony is every bit as big, multifaceted, vexing, and intractable a problem as crime is for the police chief, or world peace for the President of the United States. Only a glutton maddened by suffering and frustration can seriously believe that anyone can tell him simply what to do, or that he simply can do it himself — let's say by simply embracing some two-bit diet.

Of course, as said at the outset, one could tell the glutton: "Eat less. Eat much less. Forever. That will do it." But that would be like saying that what we need is world peace. It is true, but meaningless. It would be like saying, destroy all weapons and there will be peace. Or, distribute all the food evenly and there will be no hunger. None of these "problems" can be solved or even alleviated head-on, if only because like gluttony, they are not problems but <u>conditions</u>.

One of the greatest weaknesses of the glutton is that, without realizing it, be *believes in magic,* and regards the mountebank who promises him slimness without personality change as the prestidigitator who can turn the trick of making him savor delicious food in Falstaffian quantities forever while "pounds melt away." Does he really believe

71

there is such a guru or such a diet? Yes, he really believes that — his wish is so great as to be the father of such a ridiculous thought. Yet, underneath all these delusions there remains hidden a nagging doubt — the glutton reading, rejecting, discussing, trying, abandoning, sticking to, cursing, praising a hundred diets — has an inkling that none of them can keep what they promise and that, if he wants to become a "normal" eater of "normal" weight for the rest of his life, he must give up — *not* food — but his gluttony. He can eat anything he wants as long as he learns not to *want* too much. We cannot say it too often: Greed, not food, is the glutton's adversary. To battle gluttony by going on a diet is like playing tennis with a ball-point pen. Absurd.

The glutton does not like to hear this. But as he is ambivalent in his attitude to food — loving and hating it at the same time — he is able to mobilize his dormant dislike of his affliction. He is able to mothball his gluttony at first and then dissolve it. It is this ambivalence toward his beloved food, this forever present but at first feeble countervailing force against his appetite, that can save him.

## XIV.  *VORO ERGO SUM?*

Rene Descartes, the French philosopher of the 17th century, made himself immortal by speaking these three words:  *Cogito ergo sum*  –  I think, therefore I am.

Apparently, Descartes had suffered some existential doubts before that; and being a philosopher, he regarded the business of cogitation as so important as to prove existence.  Could it be that the glutton, consciously or not, regards eating as equally central to life?  In which case Descartes' dictum, changed into *Voro ergo sum*  –  I devour, therefore I am  –  would express what the glutton really feels.  To <u>devour</u> comes from the same root as voraciousness, and signifies a greedy and violent form of eating.  One step removed from it is the actual act of swallowing, which in Latin is *glutire*, which in turn is the origin of the word glutton/gluttony.  So, the glutton might even say: *Glutto, ergo sum,* proving his existence by the act of swallowing food.

This look at the word "glutton" makes the phenomenon of overeating illuminating.  It shows that the aim of the glutton is only secondarily to savor good food, but primarily to swallow, to fill himself up.  This would appear to be an even sadder compulsion than to be a slave to one's taste buds.   One must suspect that ultimately, albeit unconsciously, only the act of gluttony relieves the glutton from doubts that he is really alive in a real world. If this be so, it would show how thoroughly the glutton would have to change to liberate himself from his gluttony.

This writer has a friend from his Army days who is what one might call a "pure" glutton. Tall, heavyset, good natured and intelligent, he likes to eat large quantities of food. And he is not choosy. We asked him once whether it would bother him if he had only frankfurters to eat. He said it would not bother him one bit, so long as he got enough of them. One could say that his case is one of "pure" gluttony, akin to the "pure" alcoholism of some people who do not care what they drink  —  rotgut or Roederer Crystal  —  so long as they get enough alcohol into their system.

Such cases of "pure" gluttony seem to be comparatively rare. Most gluttons wrap their addiction into a blanket of gormandize  —  they don't just want food or drink but "good" food or even "great" food. But gluttony wrapped in gormandize is still just another variant of gluttony: The glutton, too  —  if no fancy dishes were available to him on occasion  —  would rather *stuff* on franks than abstain from food at mealtime.

# XV.  THE FRONTAL ATTACK

The frontal attack on his gluttony must be used to help the glutton to get started on his new life. It can be waged with an invocation in the struggle between himself and his food. When faced with the temptation of overeating, the glutton can pause. He can say to himself: "I want this food. I want it badly. But if I eat it, it will not satisfy. It may assuage my immediate craving but it will do nothing for my anxiety, frustration, greed, unhappiness. Nothing at all. It can't outlast the things that plague me so badly. It can only aggravate them. The price I will pay for eating this food will be high. It will be my bad conscience, my displeasure with myself, and the burden of being overweight."

Then he can say: "I'm not a slave to my appetite. I'm not a slave to this piece of cake. It is no small sacrifice not to eat this cake, it requires much fortitude. But I have a lot of fortitude. I've had a trying life and have overcome many things. I can overcome my craving for this too, especially since I know it will not satisfy, and more — it will make me feel badly about myself."

Often this plea with oneself will fail, obviously. If it were as easy as all that to overcome the urge to overeat, nobody would overeat. But if the formula is repeated frequently, with conscious attention to its content, it will leave a residue in the mind and soul and eventually gains power and dynamic. It is a potent mantra. The effect it can have will depend on many factors contributing to a particular individual's eating problems.

There is another way of attacking one's gluttony frontally, which is to skip an occasional meal altogether, or to try to do so. Even if this cannot be accomplished, the cosmic insistence with which the glutton's entire psychosomatic system may demand the meal will be educational for the glutton: it will show him the size of the "monster within" he is battling, its power and its wiles. (Like many alcoholics, many gluttons will say: "I can take it or leave it!" That's what they think!)

It is important to understand that gluttony is, among other things, a wily monster. It is this because of the insidious fashion in which the whole phenomenon of overeating operates. Obviously, a single serving of rich food, a single second helping, a single vast meal even, cannot and does not make a difference. At the same time, paradoxically, it makes all the difference in the world. It can be and often is, like nothing else, that comprehensible yet incomprehensible added quantity we call "the straw that breaks the camel's back."

We cannot imagine that a straw can break a camel's back under any circumstances. Yet we also know that any camel must have a breaking point which, when reached, could be exceeded by a very small weight – probably. In some way, whereas a morsel of food has no effect to the ordinary eater, it can be, for the glutton, the straw that breaks the camel's back. <u>In fact, the glutton is forever caught in the position of the camel so overburdened as not to tolerate any additional load, no matter how small</u>. The solution to this paradox is that a particular morsel of food or an entire rich meal cannot be judged as being either important or unimportant *in vacuo*. For the non-glutton it is unimportant, for the glutton it is important. But his gluttony, which tends to whisper to him half the time anyway that he is not a glutton, whispers to him that this little piece surely will not do anything bad for him because the process of gaining or losing weight is so long and gradual. But that is just a self-serving wile on the part of the glutton's devilish gluttony.

The glutton, when trying to skip a meal, must proceed in an experimental and patient frame of mind, so that he will not blame or execrate himself if he fails, or become otherwise exasperated. He also would do well to observe and register his every thought and reaction when he has decided that he will skip dinner some evening – the nature and course of the struggle, whether victorious or ending in defeat, and the thoughts it produced in his mind.

Also, the overeater must try to revise his views as to what constitutes a reasonable amount of food. What is a reasonable amount? The glutton invariable overestimates it. Seeing a slim person enjoy a chocolate malted or wolfing down a huge roast beef sandwich on rye with plenty of Russian dressing, the glutton thinks the slim man is eating "everything" all the time.

But that, of course, is not the case. That slim man may just have been grabbing the malted for energy before some arduous task, or wolfing down that sandwich because he skipped breakfast. In any event, he does not eat that way regularly.

A related phenomenon: Alcoholics also misjudge what social drinking is and how much social drinkers consume. A martini or two before dinner, then wine with the food, and some liqueur afterwards seem like social doses to them. But of course they are not, and the true social drinker will not have that quantity as a rule.

It is not possible to say what is a normal amount of food, nor is that necessary. The glutton, though emotionally immature, is, after all, no child. Even though he will like to argue the point, just in order to stymie us, he knows for himself what a normal amount of food at one sitting, or for one week, would or should be.

Gluttony can only be successfully attacked by a pincer movement. One pincer must be the frontal, direct attack; the other the deeper, more indirect effort to change personality altogether by new insight. Diets can never work because they represent the frontal attack, which alone can never succeed any more than cloth can be cut with one shear of the scissors.

# XVI.

## THE GLUTTON MUST LEARN
## TO MAKE CHANGES

## XVI . THE GLUTTON MUST LEARN TO MAKE CHANGES

The writer hopes the reader has not tried to sneak a look at these pages before reading the first part of this book. If he has, in the impatience that is so characteristic of him, and in the childish belief that somebody can just hand him some easy rules, he won't have learned any understanding of the plague that ails him. The first part of the book must be read and pondered first. The glutton can only then work on the overt changes he must make.

As a first exercise, the glutton should change as many big or little things in his life as he can before he initiates the major changes required to dissolve his gluttony. He must loosen the carapace of rituals and habits with which he encapsulates and supports himself and his affliction.

If, for example, he shaves before brushing his teeth, he can now brush his teeth before shaving. He can read his newspaper before breakfast if he usually reads it afterwards. He can take a different route to the office. He must "loosen up."

He can change his habits of talking and listening — talking less if he is a talker, or more if he is not. He can listen more instead of being inattentive, or cut people short if he generally listens to too much nonsense. He can make changes in his attire. He can stop using four-letter words if he is addicted to them, or use one occasionally if he is not. He can go to movies instead of watching TV, take a walk instead of playing golf, see people he would otherwise not see, stop seeing people he sees all the time.

He can, to speak symbolically, begin getting out of bed on the other side.

The possibilities are limitless. Naturally, many of the things he can change at once are only surface changes. From there to defeating the "dragon within" is a long way. But he may as well come to terms with the fact that it is a long way. And all changes in his daily routines will make that easier. And changing his thinking habits will help him attain control over his mind. It will help him change his moods, so that his unhappiness will be reduced, and his feelings of genuine love will increase.

Thereby, he will automatically also reduce his craving for food, his lust for food, and his slavery to food.

<u>The glutton must learn to find a new attitude to food by finding a new attitude to himself.</u>

He must learn to see food from a different perspective. This is far more than is required from the abstaining alcoholic who simply can say: "I have no power over alcohol," and leave it at that. The glutton cannot do that. He must eat. In fact, more than once a day he must encounter and cross swords with what was his enemy. He cannot say: "I'm powerless over food.: He <u>must</u> attain power over food.

How can he do it?

He must step outside himself and say a mantra that will help him: "If I had power and control over food, how would I feel about a person who does not? How would I feel about a person who spends half his waking hours either savoring or fighting food, who wrestles with food and the thought of food like Laokoon with the serpent? What would I feel for such a person? I wouldn't feel admiration but rather pity for him, for he is a pitiful creature and pity is something I, too, don't relish to be on the receiving end of. Actually, I would regard him and his pernicious passion as quite ridiculous. And ridicule is another thing I wouldn't want to be the target of. I would also regard him as a very weak person. Not so much in lacking "will power" — that does not apply here — but a weak person all around. A person too weak to confront and lead his life in such a way as to not need all that gratification and consolation that food represents for him. In sum, I would look upon him as a failure.

And he labors forever under the burden of his vice, and seems unable to shed his false perceptions as to what ails him."

This train of thought may at first depress the overeater.

But it may also help him change his perspective.

ONE:  The glutton must risk personality changes.

He must do this, not by climbing the Himalayas or driving in the Grand Prix of Monza, but in his personal relations.  Especially in his relations with himself.

Psychologists make much of the fact that people have a self-image which controls their thoughts and actions. Whether this self-image is the result of what Freud called the super-ego or was otherwise instilled in people by their parents or the entire course of their lives, or even by fate, they have a certain image of themselves and they hardly ever try to change it.  When they do try, they are usually unsuccessful at first, because their self-image is so set.  Besides, they fear to change it, for fear of actually losing themselves.

The glutton fears change doubly, since he is such a fearful person to begin with. Moreover, he thinks he cannot change himself because in the one area where he has tried so long and hard to change, namely in not being a glutton, he has indeed always failed. But there is a big difference between trying to change a trait or discarding a habit, and changing the whole person.

On the surface it would seem that the former should be easier than the latter, but that is not so. Of course, for many reasons, people do not <u>want</u> to change their whole person. They would rather get rid of a single trait or habit. It is for this reason that the offices of psychiatrists all over the world are full of people who want the doctor to free them of one single trait or weakness that bothers them, be it stuttering, blushing, various forms of impotence, shyness, a twitch, drug addiction, or even gluttony. But the psychiatrist is powerless to help them if they persist in their basic attitude to themselves.

Unlike the mechanic who can install a new carburetor and leave the rest of the car as it was before, the human psychosomatic entity is not screwed together with exchangeable or replaceable components. The human being is a whole and in a constant state of flux. At every moment, everything in a person's body and soul works together in mysterious fashion.

As a result, people are mortally afraid of changing, and the word "mortally" is used here advisedly. Their fear is in part based on the widely-held feeling that it is easier to deal with the devil one does know (in this case, oneself) than with the devil one does not know (in this case, the person one might become).

Fear of change is also based on the fear that if one changes fundamentally into something one was not before, one cannot change back if one wanted to. This is probably true, and it is where the spirit of adventure is required that we mentioned before.

But the greatest fear and resistance against changing may come from yet another corner. If the old "I" should really change in significant ways, the old "I" would be literally dead. It would be extinct. It − or "I" − would no longer exist. Which means that to change fundamentally means to die. Yet that death of the old "I" is needed, and once dead, it will be replaced by another "I," one that is easier to carry.

Such radical transformation is needed because gluttony, like other vices but even more so, is a character deformation, a character neurosis. Without a change of character, all efforts at battling gluttony would be in vain. Or, if technically successful in losing weight, as the result of an iron will, the glutton's life in self-denial will never be a happy one. Who has not seen an abstaining alcoholic at a cocktail party, chin set and eyes straight forward, his face a mask of determination but also of woe? And a glutton cannot achieve even this state of desperate abstention because – this cannot be stressed too often – he must keep eating to stay alive. And be re-stimulated.

Thus, for him to stand in front of a mirror every morning, or before a crowd like the AA members, and say "I am a glutton – I have no power over food," would be absurd.

There is one more reason why self-images tend to be almost immutable, other than the grave fears we have named. It is that the self-image is in itself a habit – in the case of the glutton a pernicious habit. His self-image is in itself his vice, or can be. Within the confines of that self-image people give themselves labels, and by doing so reinforce the traits they think they are stuck with. "I am a poor speaker," they say, or, "I'm hopeless with figures," or, "I'm not popular with the opposite sex." And if they fear they are they will be.

Of course, self-given labels not only reinforce certain traits and are very discouraging – they also serve a positive function: The person does not have to test himself any further in the areas in which he has applied the negative label to himself. Thus, the self-image is firmly anchored in a person's mind and soul for so many reasons he will find it very hard changing it but not impossible! But he must change his self-image if he wants to change his habits.

Changing one's self-image is easier for people who are afflicted by things that are less fundamental and all-pervading than gluttony. The fight against gluttony requires that the whole self-image be changed. That requires radical psychic transformation.

To undertake the task of altering his self-image, the glutton must first inventory it. He can say, first and foremost: "I am an overeater, food has power over me, and I hate that." But there are other things that will probably be true: "I am an egotist." Of course, to some extent everybody is an egotist. But the glutton is more so by several degrees. Yet he need not say to himself, I am more of an egotist than the average person. It is quite sufficient for him to say: I am an egotist. He will know what he means.

What else is he?

He is a bit of a coward. He is bored and therefore boring. He is greedy in all respects. He is a poor lover and a worse loser. He is not straightforward. He is all these and many more things which he should dredge out of his soul. This self-inventorying is not to be an exercise in mental self-flagellation and self-humiliation. The glutton must also dredge out his countervailing positive qualities, which will be listed below, and of which he may have many more than he is even aware of. This inventorying then, is not an occasion for false modesty; it is an occasion for honesty. Not "ruthless honesty," which really is more of a pose, but probing honesty, an arduous stock-taking to which one will want to add as one goes along.

The glutton should then try to change the balance of his traits by adding new positive qualities to his repertory. For example, if he is a poor listener and knows it, he can begin to think of himself as a good listener and thereby become one. At least he can make efforts in that direction.

As for his numerous bad traits, he can gradually try to <u>infiltrate</u> the past tense into his awareness of them. Instead of saying, "I am a coward," he can say: "I was a coward." Will that help? Why not try it?

<u>TWO: The glutton must learn to change his moods.</u>

Most people think that they (and also others) have no control over their moods. Wrong! Negative moods, strange as it may seem, are also a habit, just as certain ways of thinking are. This means they are man-made and can be man-altered. If a person is depressed for a specific reason or simply "blue out of the blue," he can short-circuit his depression or other negative moods by an act of will. This does not mean a person can or should be forever in aggressively good spirits. Such a person would be a great pain in everybody's neck. Even with regard to positive moods, moderation is in order. But immoderate or overly long-lasting negative moods are unwholesome. They attack a person in his weakest area and they make the glutton eat even more.

A wise yogi has said that chronic overeating is a sign that "people have given up." And of course chronic negative moods lead to giving up. Such moods can be kept from taking over, though they cannot and need not be banned from ever occurring. The Baghavad Ghita can teach you how to replace a bad mood with a good one.

THREE: The glutton must learn to change his thinking patterns.

The glutton will not be preached to here on the virtues of Positive Thinking but instead reminded of something quite different. Whether Norman Vincent Peale was right or wrong with his opinion that positive thinking yields positive results, it is true that negative thinking produces negative results. But people can control their train of thought to some extent.

To the yogis, control of the mind is the *summum bonum*. Our mind, rather than our situation, is apt to be a brutal and exhausting task master. The Baghavad Ghita calls the mind *"cittam,"* which is, transliterated, "ape" or "monkey," because the mind chatters ceaselessly, whether a person is alone or in company, riding alone to work or traveling in a crowded airplane, even while reading this book or listening to other people. The chattering of the mind can drive people crazy and it often does.

How can the mind be silenced or made immobile to the point where it becomes our servant rather than our master? This is what the yogis say we can and must achieve to lead the good life. While, for the glutton, it only means easy mastery over food.

First of all, the mind must be seen for what it is: an instrument that is not all that glorious or grandiose. This is hard for Western, "rational" man to accept. He thinks of the mind as the finest of God's creations, and as the force that is in control. Of course, the mind can be a very fine instrument, and he who can use his mind well will reap many benefits. But it is and remains an instrument, a servant; and he who lets it rave on aimlessly and endlessly as is the unbridled mind's wont, will suffer from it.

For the mind, if not carefully controlled and used by it owner rather than being in control of its owner, is intolerable, nagging, scattered, aggressive, and destructive, like a bad child running rampant.

There is a curious element in gluttony and all other vices: they pacify the mind temporarily. The drunk, though abandoning himself to unattainable fantasies, nevertheless escapes the nagging of his mind while he is drunk, as does the glutton who with his food appeases, first, his entire sensorium and, second, also his mind. In fact, he does so quite physically, by drawing blood to his stomach, away from his brain, whose insufferable chatterings and urgings become less sharp or accusing as a result. However, the glutton does not attain any control over his mind any more than any other sinner by his eating. He just dulls it and it will bounce back.

To gain control over his mind, the glutton must first come to believe that he can do so. He can do that by <u>meditating</u> on the mind and what it does or can (and cannot) do for him. He can sit in a chair and look out the window and make himself feel that the mind is not all that important, that the mind can, pleasurably, be deactivated, at least for spells of time. He can, in conversation, switch consciousness form his mind which bombards him blindly with what <u>he</u> will say next, to his heart (quite literally to his heart region) and feel what the other person is all about, why he talks, what he wants, what animates him.

92

These are useful exercises that have nothing directly to do with the control of gluttony, but will help lead there. The person who has learned how to control his mind will be less frustrated by fewer things. He will be less agitated. And it is frustration, and agitation in particular, that drives the glutton to eat.

A person can also keep his mind from thinking itself out of control about the things that irritate or depress him. This is not the same as the mood control we talked about. It is, rather, a way of aborting certain trains of thought that are either not necessary or not useful at the time they occur. The mind's thoughts can simply be rejected and exchanged for something else, much as one can reject a troublesome topic of conversation begun by someone and exchange it for a different topic. The greedy mind can be switched to things other than food if we learn to control it.

## FOUR:   The glutton must acquire discipline.

Due to the many things that plague him, the glutton is not a disciplined person. Spoiled people (and he spoils himself) rarely are. A disciplined person's self-discipline is almost automatic. It's like walking, which could also be difficult if it wasn't learned and practiced early on.

Earlier we said that the normal eater has no problem with food; he is not tempted to consume more than is good for him. This may not apply in all cases; there may also be people who, though not gluttons, are tempted to eat too much, just as others may quite often be tempted to drink too much, but deny themselves these extravagances with relative ease.

How can one attain discipline in all things? The best way is to first acquire one particular discipline. In this connection, yoga — one of the finest discipline builders -- again comes to mind. It is tailor-made for the overeater in every respect. It imparts to the practitioner an increasing power over himself, a steadily growing self-control in all areas of life, including one's eating. It also reduces his anxiety, which is one of the great promoters of over-eating.

Finally, by greatly enhancing a person's oxygen intake, yoga makes him calmer, wiser, and less greedy. In fact, just to breathe deeply in moments of stress or, better yet, as a regular habit, will have the same beneficial results, albeit on a reduced scale. In fact, when struggling against that piece of cake, simply taking a deep breath or two may produce glorious victory.

Unfortunately, there are almost as many quacks in the area of yoga as there are in weight reduction, so, *caveat emptor!* Our country abounds with little old ladies who take handsome fees from people to sit cross-legged in groups and chant. But that is not yoga. Yoga can only be learned from a true yogi, and only by private instruction. This is not expensive, as yoga can be learned in about 20 sessions at least to the point from which it can be effectively practiced and further developed by the practitioner himself. At that point, books on yoga can help, though they cannot help at all if a person does not take private lessons first.

The benefit of yoga for the glutton is, finally, that it reshapes his body while he is losing weight due to his new way of life. It makes him feel better. And to feel better reduces all morbid appetite for food.

FIVE:  The glutton must develop pride.

So far the word "pride" has not yet been used, even though it is connected with much that was talked about. Language wisely distinguishes between pride and false pride, and between pride and vanity. Of vanity the glutton has more than his share. But in order to overcome his weakness for and dependance on food, he must develop true pride.

Pride – like vice – is an old-fashioned word. One can search modern texts in psychiatry or psychology in vain for it. Yet, it is a word that exists and has existed for a very long time in every Western language (and presumably in other languages as well). It represents a quality without which men cannot lead good and sensible lives despite the fact – or perhaps because of the fact – that there is something abrupt, harsh, even unreasonable about it.

But pride is a many splendored thing and a great simplifier. People will tell you, usually with genuine satisfaction, that they did something, or refrained from doing something, simply because they were too proud to do otherwise. They do not say that they analyzed the situation down to the last iota, or made every last ounce of effort to resolve it. Instead of hanging on for dear life, they just quit pursuing something that troubled their self-esteem, their sense of pride, or did something that made them proud.

Often pride will lead to a negative act, i.e., to abandon or "sacrifice" something. And more often than not it will not even be a rational decision. But almost always it will be a right decision, unless the person making it is a fool. Pride and its assertion is closely associated with freedom, and it always helps attain some freedom. Quite possibly, the spurned suitor could have wheedled his way into his Dulcinea's good graces or even her bed if he had kept debasing himself and showering her with diamonds. Quite conceivably, the ambitious employee could have obtained that junior partnership if he had continued to kowtow to an unreasonable boss.

But they didn't, and their lives and loves are the better for it, no matter what they seem to have given up. More often than not, they did not even give up anything, as their craven pursuit would not have been rewarded anyway.

Pride told them no longer to submit to the abuse or tribulations others put in their way of obtaining certain objectives. On a more fundamental level, they decided no longer to submit to the tribulations which their own desires for those objectives imposed on them — the tribulations and the humiliations. They became too tired to stumble on from defeat to defeat; and though they neither fully explored the situation nor rationally resolved it, they simply cut it short and forgot about it.

The quality of pride allows a person to put down his foot abruptly, regardless of whether there seems any hope left of success. If a person cannot cast out a desire for something that is too highly priced in terms of self-esteem, he or she is in a bad way indeed. For life is full of desirable things that humiliate those who pursue them too long and ardently. People cannot have most of the things they desire. If they have pride, they have the ability to put a stop to an intolerable and humiliating situation. They can commit instant surgery. They have a weapon at their command that is not only powerful but unique in the arsenal of man who must make his way through life in a labyrinth of unattainable objectives and unfulfilled desires.

The glutton, too, must at some point reach a state of mind in which he simply is too proud to be mastered by food and the desire for or thought of food, or the concern with his weight or shape.

This may seem to be in some conflict with what was said before, which was that the glutton must go very far into analyzing and comprehending this affliction before he can free himself from it. But there is no contradiction here. The point is that the secret of success against so formidable and tricky an enemy as gluttony can only be a mixed arsenal of every conceivable weapon, used in orchestration. Self-analysis, if deep and courageous and insistent enough, will be an essential weapon in the battle. Pride is what will help the glutton wage his with success.

After all, a person who is so addicted to the caresses of a substance on his tongue and palate or a "satisfying" feeling in his belly that he is enthralled, mastered, and in fact mocked and humiliated by it, is not an admirable person, especially if he wants to but cannot get out of his predicament. And simple pride can come to his aid when a frontal attack is called for. Against all the other childish accouterments of gluttony as well, the constant weighing, the constant reading and talking about foods and diets, the constant celebrations as to what he will have for lunch or dinner, simply pride is a powerful and necessary antidote. The glutton, after a penetrating look at his entire human condition, <u>can</u> say: TO HELL WITH IT, I SIMPLY WILL NO LONGER PUT UP WITH THIS NONSENSE. Unless he can do this, he is not likely to succeed.

Just as no diet can keep the glutton from feeling empty and hungry no matter how loudly the reducing quacks swear they can provide such a diet, no amount of analysis and self-comprehension can keep the glutton from having to make some hard decisions at times, decisions he must make abruptly, without much thinking, out of pride.

This is very hard for the glutton to do as he is accustomed to spoiling himself and because his pride is impaired from way back. Indeed, his pride largely accounts for his greed and perennially wounded ego and vanity, and thus his gluttony. Fortunately for him, contrary to incurable psychopaths or sociopaths, the glutton generally <u>did</u> have pride as a child, so pride <u>is</u> still in him and can do its share. It is just that his innate pride was so badly mishandled, stymied, and subdued by later experiences that he can no longer feel it except as a gnawing discomfort and reproach. But he has it — probably in ample measure. If he can liberate it, activate it, and deploy it on his field of battle, he will be on his way.

The glutton, too, though he sometimes may feel with bitterness that he isn't, is a child of God and part of this world — a fact from which he may derive some satisfaction and pride. Conversely, he should consider that no matter how withdrawn and isolated his gluttony has made him, he can be a "self-made man." God (or nature, or fate) has given him his body only in trust and on loan, so to speak, and he has a certain obligation to feed it properly and keep it in good shape. This thought, too, should help him.

SIX:   The glutton must learn to transfer his voraciousness.
Freud talked a great deal about sublimation. The ability to sublimate is one of the most important factors in the civilization and socialization of man. Without it, men would still be savages, living in caves and following only their most primitive drives and instincts.

This, incidentally, does not mean, at least not in the mind of this author, that such a state of affairs would be "bad," nor that it would be "good," either morally or from the point of view of human happiness or fulfillment. We do not know whether primitive man hunting and devouring game was happier or unhappier than the squash-playing, big city executive or the inhabitants of the social register. The point here is only that we live at present in a world that, for want of a more accurate description, we call civilized, and so be it.

Now, we say that the world has mostly come about because of man's drive and ability to sublimate. Every reader is familiar with the simple meaning of the term: than an inclination to cut up people can be sublimated into surgery which saves lives and relieves suffering instead of inflicting it. Or that the desire to kill or to fight can be sublimated into selfless heroism on the battlefield. Or that the infantile desire to smear excrement on the walls can be sublimated into painting beautiful paintings.

In other words, where deep-seated and destructive urges cannot be eliminated, they can be given different and "higher" aims, i.e., sublimated. When pursued in the new direction, even in a creative way, they may still do a certain amount of harm to him who pursues them and the people around him. For example, a workaholic can also do damage to himself and others. But, except in extreme cases, a workaholic does less harm to himself and his family than an alcoholic. And he often creates wealth and other goods in the process. A compulsive reader, worker, golfer, competitor, or chess player will – rightly – arouse our concern, but not as much as a compulsive eater, drinker, or drug user.

In the glutton, his voraciousness is generally so primal and deep-seated that he cannot hope to get rid of it easily or quickly; it must be sublimated, i.e., transformed into something more benign. A more contemplative attitude, as will be discussed in the next chapter, can help but it can only help; it cannot do the job as it needs to be done. The glutton is therefore advised to try to transfer his ingrained voraciousness to targets other than cheese, meat, gravy, and pie. He also could condition himself to "devour" books instead. That would be an instance of sublimation. And a relief for him.

All of life is a multifarious intake and output. A person goes on a trip where he "takes in" the sights and sounds of another land (with the "appetite" for it varying from traveler to traveler), and then tells or writes about it. Not long ago a dying friend told this author he could no longer enjoy reading because his reading was, in the main, preparation and substance for his own writing, and his writing days were over.

In other words, people take in, transform, and put out all the time. Those who do so in a restrained cycle and in sensible proportion between physical, intellectual, and spiritual matter, are fortunate indeed. Most unhappiness in the world is caused by disproportion among these areas.

The act of creating anything is always one of creatively transforming input into output. The writer, the architect, the financier, the teacher, the painter, even the lowly employee, cannot do "his thing" without first absorbing, learning (we often call it), or saturating himself with feelings, impressions, data. The glutton also saturates himself but he does so with food, which he transforms only into feces, the Latin word for "things done" or output.

This is a sorry state of affairs if practiced in excess and in disproportion to other input-transformation-output cycles of which the glutton, too, being a human being, is intrinsically capable. Yet it does not occur to him that a book, or all sorts of other things, can be as delicious as a dish made of the finest lobster, or a Grade A goose liver flown in directly from Perigord; that, in fact, a book can be devoured too. Many readers devour books and set the input-transformation-output cycle into motion. This is not desirable but better than devouring food.

The glutton can also transfer his voraciousness, albeit in reduced measure, to other targets: He can ingest exquisite art in museums. He can listen to music, play chess, or become a good conversationalist. He can become an avid listener to what others have to say, a posture not often practiced by the glutton. The glutton can even begin to partake in the joys of sex. For sex can be fun! Unfortunately, the glutton often has trouble in that department, so much so that he may have given up on sex, more or less, except in his desires and fantasies. In fact, as already stated, his trouble with sex is likely to be a contributing cause to his gluttony.

We see something interesting here: the voraciousness for food that drives the glutton, and that is caused in part by sexual or other frustrations, is not the same primitive and direct voraciousness that drives the infant toward food, but is a _displacement_ and _substitution_. Thus, having re-targeted his voraciousness once before from desires for sex and or other gratifications, such as vanity, desire for wealth, and so on, to his beloved food, why can the glutton not re-target his voraciousness a second time, toward non-material, or at least, non-fattening targets?

One more word here on the subject of sex. Aside from the fact that the glutton generally suffers from certain types of sexual dysfunction, he generally will also bring the same attitude toward it as toward food, namely a certain voraciousness, with heavy emphasis on quantity, i.e., promiscuity and less on love and affection. But sex without love tends to be frustrating. It consequently gives the overeater one more source of frustration that in turn feeds his gluttony. Obviously, sexual voracity divorced from love causes much suffering to those so afflicted. How this can be cured has mostly remained a riddle. However, as with everything else, to be conscious of it can help the sex-starved as much as would the trimmer figure and keener look the glutton would acquire if he ate less.

Whether the glutton can re-target his voraciousness, and what targets he will select, will be to some extent the result of experimentation. He therefore should experiment with every possible input-transformation-output cycle until he finds one or several that suit him. The cycle will allow him to sublimate some of his voraciousness into other channels than eating food and creating feces.

SEVEN:   The glutton must learn not to be so unhappy.

Just as oysters are an acquired taste, happiness is also largely acquired. Not an acquired taste precisely, but an acquired habit or posture. It rarely comes about by itself. This may be one reason why people are so anxious to fall and be in love: if reciprocated, the in-loveness will produce instant and complete happiness, regardless of what other factors assault the blissful lovers.

105

As far as happiness is concerned, America is the most curious of countries. People talk and think about happiness all the time. It was even written into the Constitution that its pursuit was an inalienable right. Gluttons (and others) would do well, however, to accept the bitter fact that the Constitution does not regard happiness itself as an inalienable right but only its pursuit, which is a different pigeon altogether.

American pursue happiness with such a vengeance, that the thought occurs that they must be the unhappiest people in the Western world. For no one who is happy would make such a fuss over its pursuit.

It is interesting here to consider television commercials. The people on the screen drinking Pepsi or Lite Beer, washing dishes with Cascade, polishing their floors with Product A, baking their cakes with Product B, deodorizing their bathrooms with Product C, or riding around in roadster D all have one thing in common: they are all ordinary folk, and they are all happy.

They are all healthy, too. They get along great with their children, partners, or bosses. They have not a problem in the world, unless it is what juice to buy or what cat litter to select. Even though clearly not rich, they never seem to have money cares. All young, apparently successful, and — above all — obviously radiantly happy.

And the glutton feels left out and envies them. That the reality is otherwise, everybody (and especially the glutton) should know. After all, excessive and ludicrous demands are being made on almost everyone in our reality. There is never enough money to pay all the bills, let alone to do all the things one wants to do. One's health is no better than just okay. Relations with children, parents, bosses, partners are full of aggravation and friction. Time passes too quickly, opportunities are missed, bad investments are made, wrong choices (especially after much deliberation and agonizing) are commonplace.

In addition, there is much cultural malaise, existential anxiety, fear of the future and distress over the present. The house may be burglarized, the children abducted. War may break out. Times in general are bad in one way or another, it seems, and getting worse. Marriages go sour. Painful loss is inevitable. Death looms, then strikes.

The suffering to which man is heir in his little life is deep indeed, and springs from a seemingly inexhaustible well. What words can describe the pains of unrequited or lost love? What words encompass the agony of the slights, rejections, losses, pains that come anyone's way, year in and year out?

Though he likes to appear and comport himself as strong and serene, American man — not all but most — is endowed with a soul as sensitive as a butterfly. (Much more than a Frenchman's, for example). That soul gets mistreated in his childhood by his equals, his teachers, his elders and, yes, most often by one or both of his parents. To long without avail for a better life is man's constant lot; sorrow and distress his daily bread.

There are, for the well-adjusted, some happy hours and days, but they are not abundant. They are so rare as to be well remembered. Happiness is a flighty sprite; suffering a faithful, unshakable companion.

Small wonder man needs all the consolation he can get. But true consolation is hard to come by. And, to close the vicious circle, the dearth of available consolation is one reason why there is so much pain and why it is so great and enduring.

To add to man's distress, there are many sources of false consolation. Gluttony is perhaps the most prominent among them, next to alcohol. Food, liquor and drugs are the great pseudo-consolers, the great diverters and deadeners in our lives. They only deaden, generally; they do not kill. This means that what they deaden rises to the surface again, like a rock that was covered only momentarily by the flooding waves but emerges again when they recede.

The glutton will not accept that it is man's lot on earth to suffer more than to enjoy, to be sad more often than to be happy. This stubborn non-acceptance of his adds immeasurably to his travail. Like Tantalus, who must forever roll his heavy stone back up the mountain every time he nears the top, the glutton holds on to the causes of his agonies instead of working them through. And he suffers more than others.

How, then, can one be happy? What is happiness?

It is a curious feature of the English language that, contrary to German or French, it distinguishes between "happy" and "lucky." Although a <u>lucky</u> fellow who just won the lottery has reason to be <u>happy</u>, the two terms are different. One refers to a state of mind, the other to a fortunate accident.

In German the word is *Glueck*, which means both luck and happiness. In English, as in German, the word was originally the same for happy and lucky, in that the word <u>happy</u> comes from the word <u>happen</u>. This would seem to indicate that the state of happiness is at best occasional and transitory, "happening" only on special occasions when something good and unexpected <u>happens</u> to make us <u>happy</u>.

But Americans aspire to a <u>state</u> of happiness, i.e., a continuing condition which, even by the word's definition, is not in the cards. Especially the glutton, whose strong suit is wishing but whose weak suit is willing, dreams of happiness. And the more he dreams of happiness, the unhappier he becomes and the more he eats.

No doubt the pursuit of happiness (and does the word <u>pursuit</u> not warn us of its elusiveness?) can be one of the most powerful and permanent sources of unhappiness. The poor glutton who must endure all the unhappiness his fellow men also endure must, on top of that, endure the unhappiness over his being forever unhappy about his weight and his insatiable greed.

As acute unhappiness is the glutton's single most powerful impulse driving him to overeat, it is of supreme importance for him to become happier than he is. But how can he go about it?

There are, happily, two ways in which unhappiness can be reduced. One is to make things happen one wants to happen, to acquire the things one wants to have, and then to find that those were indeed the things one wanted. But few people are so "lucky" as to be able to do that. Moreover, with all things being constantly in flux, even the happy possessor of all his blessings soon starts worrying, quite rightly, about their permanence. Love, like money, like position, can easily evanesce. Still, one way to be happy is to have all one wants — a most unlikely albeit not entirely impossible "happening" in our world.

The other and more available way to attain a form of happiness is for the unhappy person to work on his unhappiness and not permit it to be so big, so all-pervading, so over-powering, so permanent. The glutton has every reason to be unhappy over his gluttony, especially if he confronts the depth of his affliction. But, even so, he need not be as unhappy over it as he tends to be, nor over anything else that disturbs or frustrates him in life. Unhappiness can be in some part a posture, if not actually a pose, played out on the stage of life before the human audience, designed by the actor to harvest sympathy and unearned privileges, and for oneself the excuse for transgressions and failures.

Then it actually pays off, though at exorbitant cost, to be unhappy. For the opportunistic unhappiness, even if partly pose or habit, is real and painful. In the case of anyone who is slave to a vice like gluttony, it is an added stimulus in the wrong direction, i.e., to eat.

Luckily, however, one can will oneself to be less unhappy even if circumstances do not change or become even worse. In the first place, one can count one's blessings. Trite and silly though that may seem, one can derive a certain reduction of unhappiness from one's blessings. Naturally, when I do not have a cold, I cannot be radiantly happy that I haven't got one, but to some extent I can. Is there one of us who has not sat in his car, profoundly unhappy over a whole combination of misfortunes and truly in a black and desperate mood, who was not jolted out of this mood when seeing a blind person grope his way across the street with a white cane? We see at such moments, in a flash, that though our unhappiness may be real and justified, we have exaggerated it, dramatized it, seen it in disproportionate, unrealistic ways. There are two reasons for our having done that. One is that, for whatever reason, many of us have acquired at least a mild masochistic trait: one of the most common vices is to feel sorry for oneself over and above the justified measure. The other reason is — and this is very different — that many of us are at least a trifle obsessional, so that a failure or loss in the particular area of our obsessiveness will make us more unhappy than is justified by circumstances, or than we would be if we looked at the situation more dispassionately.

Thus, unhappiness is capable of being reduced by sheer will and, at times, of being short-circuited altogether. Unhappiness can be "managed" and reduced. Most gluttons do not know this and therefore never try. Just as they do not know that any person can, with some practice and determination, learn to control − up to a point − his mind and his moods in general, he can learn how to control and reduce his unhappiness. He can say to himself, "WHAT IN HELL AM I SO UNHAPPY ABOUT?" and, "WHY CAN I NOT AT LEAST ENJOY THIS MOMENT?" This will do wonders for the glutton if he practices it, especially in front of a mirror. It will reduce his greed and craving, and deprive him of one of his favorite unconscious excuses to indulge his unconscionable vice.

There is one thing in urgent need of clarification here: It is not altogether accurate to say that happiness can be learned. Even people of above-average emotional vigor and maturity are rarely totally happy, except temporarily.

There is a state of non-happiness/non-unhappiness which, considering the human condition, is a desirable state of mind. Certainly it is more desirable than straight unhappiness. It is a sort of neutral domain, one which is never sung about in ballads or mentioned in our overly romantic world. It's a state in which a person is not happy, but definitely not unhappy either. Where a person feels in reasonable harmony with his world, his fellows, his expectations. Compared to the state of unhappiness, which is a state of acute suffering, this neutral state of being neither happy nor unhappy is paradise. It is a sensible and realistic frame of mind. And it requires no palliatives, such as overeating.

This state can be learned; it can be attained by repeated acts of will and self-admonitions. A person can say to himself, with emphasis and, eventually, great effect: "I certainly am not radiantly happy. But who is? And at this moment, this day, I am not unhappy. Why should I be? There are still a good many things in the works that may turn out fine."

Even if a person is desperately unhappy for a specific reason — generally over a loss that cannot be repaired — he can reach this plateau of being neither happy nor unhappy fairly quickly if he tries to and if he is satisfied with it, instead of insisting on exchanging his soul-wrenching misery at one blow for corresponding heights of ecstasy.

All great psychological suffering eventually passes, but not without mourning, which – Freud emphasized – cannot be done in a day. But it can be shortened by the victim's striving for a neutral state instead of asking fate for compensating delights for the suffering he had to endure. The state of chronic unhappiness, not caused by a particular event at a given moment, which is the overeater's basic mood, can be eliminated and replaced, in time and with practice, by a neutral feeling of being neither happy nor unhappy. By a feeling, in fact, that happiness as imagined by so many people is a childish and egotistical fantasy, which can and should be discarded – the sooner the better.

The person who is chronically unhappy, rather than "crushed" over a single event, can work his way out of that dark hole into the cool no-man's land of being neither happy nor unhappy, which will be a great and appetite suppressing improvement. Neither the person plunged into unhappiness by a single blow of fate nor the person dwelling habitually and resentfully in the netherworld of despair, should use his condition to compensate and console himself with food, as this is like jumping from the frying pan into an entire conflagration.

In his efforts to exchange unhappiness for non-happiness/non-unhappiness, the glutton should also remember that the Baghavad Ghita tells us that there is in us our innermost self, the *atman*, which always retains an imperturbable coolness and dispassionate stance, observing our joys or sorrows like a third party that is not really involved.

Instead of further alienating this already remote *atman* with food, the glutton should try to become aware of its existence inside his soul, helping his *atman* to spread the mood of detachment to his whole person. This will have a calming and consoling effect – more potent, real and lasting than the greatest culinary debauchery imaginable.

### EIGHT: The glutton must learn to "will."

Gluttons, smokers, alcoholics, and other addicts bore us with their having "no will power." They produce a sheepish grin on this occasion, as though to say, I am an honest fellow at least, or: Isn't that disarming?, or: Please tell me that you, too, have no will power.

But this is stupid. To overcome one's addictions does not take "will power," nor does it <u>not</u> take "will power." Will power is a meaningless term, suggesting that one should be able to overcome a temptation by a sheer and narrowly focused will. But as Thomas Mann has shown in his great short story, "Mario and the Magician," he who wills only negatively (in this case a callow youth on a stage trying not to succumb to a repulsive mountebank hypnotizing him) cannot hope to succeed in the long run. For to will _not_ to do something, and not to will anything at all, is the same – and impossible.

This is true for any negative decision made in the area of addiction. If I decide not to smoke this cigarette, it is not the same kind of decision it is if I decide to smoke it. For if I decide to smoke it and light it and actually smoke it, that decision is now irreversible. But if I decide not to smoke the cigarette, the same decision will stare me in the face again five minutes later, and again in five hours, and in five days.

Unless I "will" something broader and more positive than merely not to smoke, I must eventually succumb.

Quite different from the unrealistic notion of "will power" is the actual will that is inherent in people. It is of greatly varying vigor, type or effect. A person needs the will to live, otherwise he dies. If he is emotionally and otherwise in good shape, that will is strong and broad and automatically helps him overcome all hazards.

117

In the overeater and addict in general, that will to live is impaired, to the point that when deadening his consciousness with his favorite substance, he reduces rather than enhances his aliveness. In fact, he commits endlessly repeated small or/and symbolic acts of self-destruction, of suicide.

If his will to live becomes less beleaguered by his fears and negative passions, if his anxiety declines and the targets for his positive will (rather than his pallid wishing) become clearer and more varied, he also will discover, quite coincidentally, the will to resist the very food that — in a curious way — consumes _him_ while he is consuming _it_.

NINE:   The glutton must gain self-confidence.

People are always told they must have more self-confidence, which is a bore. Just as nobody is altogether free, nobody is altogether secure, and nobody has the amount of self-confidence modern self-help books prescribe, except some atypical maniacs in institutions or jails.

But there are various targets or areas of self-confidence where the glutton is particularly wanting, and where he can improve.

The overeater has no confidence that (1) he can refrain from eating more than he thinks he should, and (2) that he can exist on less food. He does not trust himself with food, and rightly so. Like the alcoholic, he is easily seduced to take the first forbidden step, and then another and another.

But the overeater also feels he simply cannot exist without excessive food. Like the alcoholic who feels that unless he has some drinks he cannot get through the night (or whatever it is he is trying the "get through" in his passivity and unfreedom), the glutton has similar feelings of non-confidence in his ability to cope with "life" unless he overeats.

The feeling of confidence  —  that he does not need excessive food to "live"  —  is hard for him to attain. But it can be acquired by resolute trial and practice.

Eventually the ability to live without stuffing himself will appear on the overeater's woefully limited horizon, on his inner screen, and it will contribute to his egress from the inferno.

## TEN:   The glutton must learn how to be free.

It is contemporary man's wont to babble forever about freedom, the Free World, his being a free man, others not being free men, and all that kind of balderdash. He blows himself up like a frog with false pride when reading *The New York Times* or watching "60 Minutes." convinced that it was worth having been driven out of paradise to enjoy such great freedom. He pities the poor slobs in China or wherever, who have no freedom and are slaves of their masters.

Well, he is not all that free either.

In the first place, there is no free man, even though man's entire history has been a vain effort to be free. Yet that effort has not been entirely vain. Compared to other ages — by no means all — we have a lot of freedoms at our disposal.

But to have a thing at our disposal is not the same as having it or using it wisely. Only if everything else is in its proper place can we take and enjoy the freedoms available to us. We then are still not free, but at least relatively free, as compared to some others, here or there.

The glutton can make no convincing claim that he is a free man. No Mao or Stalin was ever as relentless, capricious and implacable a slave driver as is gluttony or any other addictions. A man who cannot stand up to a baked potato with sour cream and chives is no more a free man than the prisoner perishing in the icy Siberian wastes. The glutton, or any other addict, does not even know what freedom is.

He is the victim of a tyranny worse than most other tyrannies, as it is of his own making and predilection. Not only is he in the clutches of his personal tyrant, but he is infatuated with him. He cannot even stand up to his torturer as the dissenter might to a dictator. But even though he does not really see it, the glutton is vaguely aware of his unfreedom, and he resents it the same way he resents almost everything else.

Fortunately, this awareness, no matter how dim, can contribute to the glutton's salvation. He can shake himself free from his passion and become at least as free a person as the human condition permits. This shows us how important every morsel of food, if consumed by the glutton against his will, really is. To the non-glutton it may seem peculiar that the glutton agonizes over eating or not eating that baked potato, but the glutton has reason to agonize: not only his girth but also his self-esteem is at stake!

Some years ago this writer was talking with an attractive, young woman who was struggling with being just a bit overweight. She was in a state of deep depression because the day before, at a wedding reception, she had eaten two pastries she had not wanted to eat. To her peers her distress seemed silly. But for her, like any lost battle, the matter was not ridiculous at all. To eat the pastries would have been as nothing for a non-glutton. But to eat those pastries against one's will, against one's great and valorous efforts, to be defeated – a human being, created in the image of God – by two pastries, is a different matter. The young woman was dejected not just by that insignificant intake of food but by her defeat, her manifest and exasperating unfreedom. Yet, she did not understand her problem. She thought in terms of "calories" rather than slavery – her slavery to food. Of course two pastries are not important. But for the glutton who first resists and then succumbs to them, they are a painful defeat.

If a glutton thought in terms of slavery, rather than calories, it would help him reform. He would attain and enjoy some of the real freedom our society provides. A further word on the young woman who lost "the battle of the pastries." She belonged to the category of persons who are not really overweight, but fear to become so, or think they already are so, in the sense that what they regard as their desirable weight is in fact what is below normal (or natural) for them and therefore impossible to attain or maintain except by constant under-eating. Such persons may be driven by vanity, or an entire upside-down view of the human condition.

### ELEVEN: The glutton must learn to love.

We have already discussed sex. Now we must talk about love. To love is fun. Not just to love another person to whom one is married, or infatuated or friends with, but to love anybody or anything at all, for whatever reason. If you see a person telling you he loves Sicily, or the people who live next door, or a book he read, or a new sweater he bought, his face will be bright and relaxed. If he tells you about a person he hated, a film he detested, a boss who offended him, his face will be grim. People want to see their man elected to office, not jut because they think he will do a better job but because then they can see and like him. It is more fun to like than to hate. There is a pleasure and harmony in loving and displeasure and disharmony in hating. Harmony feels better to the soul. And overeaters are often hidden haters.

But it is not easy to love. Especially for a person who has been hurt. And the overeater has been hurt. We cannot tell where or when or by whom; but we can tell he has been hurt badly. And he is still smarting.

In addition, he constantly hurts himself. Being very critical of himself, he tends to have a critical, severe, unloving posture to all others, including himself, and all things. He demands perfection not only of his bechamel sauce (yet finds it "right"), but also of everything else. This does not preclude that he will at the same time swoon over something or somebody unworthy, especially if that thing or person is distant and unobtainable. But he has a hard time loving anybody or anything. Least and last of all himself. And this is true no matter how much he "spoils" himself with allegedly delectable food.

Why is he so unloving? Because he is unaware of the simple fact that loving, like "cutting down" on one's unhappiness, or controlling one's mind, can actually be learned. Naturally, he need not learn to gush phonily over this or that. On the contrary. But as he has love — and unlike the psychopath, the glutton does have love — he can condition himself to let it flow. He can learn not to stifle it by his chronic anger, envy, hostility and greed.

But what or whom, he may exclaim with exasperation, should he love? He can try to love, or at least like, people in general more than he does now. At least, he can try to hate or dislike them less. This does not in the least mean he must do violence to his critical judgment. This writer knows an elderly woman who hates the superintendent of her modest building because he is "so stupid." And the man really is very stupid. But other than that he is quite a lovable old man — helpful, concerned, reliable. Why should she not love or at least like him? Because he can't converse about Emerson? She could do so without in the least surrendering her critical judgment of his wanting mental endowments.

What on earth has all that to do with me, the glutton might ask at this point with his characteristic impatience. The answer is that, as was said before, the glutton can never hope to overcome his gluttony unless he undergoes such fundamental and all-pervading changes as will make his head swim when he hears about them. So profound are the roots of his gluttony that equally profound must be the change in his nature.

Hatred, envy, anger, snobbism, unexpressed dislike (because the glutton is too timid to express them) are the principal brakes on his ability to change. At the same time these are among the most potent motors driving his gluttony. He continues to crave food as a palliative to these negative feelings, and thus keeps overeating. It all hangs together and becoming evident if the glutton will only take the time and make the effort to trace the connections.

TWELVE:  The glutton must learn to enjoy foodless conviviality.

Hard though it is for the glutton to even imagine it, some people get together and enjoy each other's company even when they are not eating. Actually, the glutton may not find this all that hard to believe when he thinks of alcoholics who get together just to drink, or of people who practice group sex, or of people who read Elizabethan poems. They do not need food, at least not for the moment.

For the glutton, by contrast every encounter is reason to celebrate with food: the meeting of an old friend, the making of a new friend, the departure or arrival of someone, the getting-together of friends for celebration or lucubration. He knows some persons enjoy each other's company without eating, such as people who go hunting, sailing, hiking, or golfing together. But that is not for him.

The glutton may be annoyed for being reminded of the fact that some people engage in foodless conviviality. In fact, he may indignantly point out that he, too, occasionally engages in such pursuits with friends. He, too, may be a hunter or golfer or chess player absorbed by such activities and the good fellowship while he is at it. But when the fun is over he finds his craving for food redoubled, letting him have it with both barrels.

Naturally, he will have to eat like everybody else. But when he meets that long-lost friend whom he has not seen since childhood, or when he meets Joe Blow whom he saw only a week ago, he does not ignore such an opportunity to overeat.

The underlying cause of such eruptions of camaraderie is that, at heart, the glutton is bored most of the time. He's bored with himself and with almost everybody else. Consequently his tendency to overeat is forever stimulated further.

But he **need** not be so bored!  Other people are at least as interesting as he is, as he would find out if he had the zip and courage to suppress his obsession with food and pay more attention to other people than merely the meals he may share with them. He then would learn something about _true_ conviviality, as distinguished from the pseudo-conviviality which we see whenever people congregate to satisfy their gluttony or any other vices that hold them in slavery.

THIRTEEN:  The glutton must learn how to cry.

Contrary to what one might think when viewing the forever jubilating Pepsi Generation on TV, our world _is_ a vale of tears.  Life is sad or trying in many respects, and full of anxious moments.

Most gluttons suffer a greater share of these than the ordinary person.  But instead of coping with them by pausing to cry or at least pause until they feel better, they run to the fridge or sit down to an outrageous meal and eat until they feel even worse.

Just as the glutton is in denial about many things, he denies the routine sadness of life. He fails to deal with it in an emotionally constructive fashion.  He batters himself and his grief with food instead of working through what must be worked through anyway.  That puts him at a disadvantage.  Others can dissolve in a few hours or days of true grief and honest tears what the glutton may carry around with himself for years. He doesn't let it surface and give it its due in tears and sadness.

This does not mean the glutton must become a sad sack and go around with a long face day in and day out. On the contrary, he must laugh, too; and the chances are he has not learned that either. When the glutton is confronted with elating or depressing experiences, he must learn to react with tears or laughter, instead of sullen silence and with an extra boost of sharpened appetite. Of course food can console – *vide* those Irish wakes. But that is not for him.

The overeater must learn how to cry, as he seems even less able to cry than to laugh. In most people's lives, reasons to cry, though they may not outweigh reasons to laugh – this is a question of temperament rather than reality – are frequent and strong. An ability to meet such occasions with tears rather than food is crucial for the glutton.

Remember, not even for one of us is life a bed of roses! And for most of us it is a bed with many thorns. To be sad, to mourn, to be dejected and discouraged is a normal state of affairs. It is wholesome and therapeutic. If the sad things in life, including the ever-present prospect of sickness and death – one's own and others' – are not dealt with in the only way in which they can be dealt with effectively — namely by quiet introspection and a few tears rather than double helpings of roast beef with all the trimmings — they cannot assume that proper place in the soul. Instead they only stimulate whatever vice a person uses as a sop in his effort at rejecting the reality of life itself.

## FOURTEEN:  The glutton must learn how to pray.

Praying is a curious occupation or habit. It has been done everywhere by people ever since the beginning of recorded history. It has been practiced by everybody, believer or not, in ordinary situations but especially in certain moments of distress, danger or despair. Whereas in our enlightened times prayers may be out of style, almost every soldier in battle has at one time or another prayed.  In an earlier age people even prayed to be helped to ward off temptation — a practice tailor-made for gluttons!

People who do not or cannot pray generally say they do not believe in God, or a just god, or a god interested in individuals, and they therefore cannot address or seek solace or fortitude in Him or him. They think and behave like people who would — quite rightly — refuse to address a petition to a non-existing authority or administration.

But praying is different from addressing a petition to the bureaucracy. Perhaps its greatest merit is that it does not require the person who prays to be religious or even a believer. This is an important aspect of prayer in our largely non-religious times.

Anyone can pray for anything at any time. Often this will be without effect, of course, or at least without the desired success. Someone praying frequently that the Dodgers should win may find that they have been clobbered, but he may also realize while praying for their victory that he is a fool for attaching such absurd importance to the game. That could be of greater value to him than if the Dodgers won! It just is not predictable what the result of prayer will be.

Ultimately, prayer is <u>concentration</u>, and concentration always helps in some ways. The glutton tends to be intellectually and emotionally diffuse; his overly heavy concentration on food causes and shows this. For food does not deserve the kind of attention the glutton devotes to it. If he concentrates on it as he does, it is a form of pseudo or ersatz concentration, interfering with <u>all</u> forms of piety. Especially when tempted by his gluttony, i.e., by the devil, prayer, silent or otherwise, it may help the glutton to prevail over the most tempting delicacies.

## FIFTEEN:   The glutton must learn how to make music.

One of the easiest and most direct — and also most civilized — ways of discharging excess emotional pressure is through music. To listen to music is regarded as therapeutic. But it is a passive posture, and passivity and the glutton's constant emotion over-pressure are a poor combination.

To make music, on the other hand, i.e., to play an instrument of whatever kind, is high activity. It requires skill, practice and complete attention while, at the same time allowing the music-maker to drain off, in fact to sublimate, his emotional excess baggage in agreeable, liberating and socially positive fashion.

Gluttony is, among so many other things, physical passivity, if not paralysis, in the epicenter of always raging emotional storms that cry to be assuaged — with food in the case of the glutton. To sublimate such feelings with any creative effort, be it writing, gardening, learning or doing any other type of work, is possible. But it is easier to do it by making music. Gluttons rarely play, be it games or instruments. If they did it would do wonders for them. No one, while playing one of his favorite tunes on his favorite instrument, has ever craved, at the same moment, food of any kind. And the displacement of emotional energy into music, rather than deadening it with food, can carry over into the entire day and beyond.

And if the food addict cannot or will not play music, at least he can sing. That, too, will curb his craving.


### SIXTEEN: The glutton must learn to recognize temptation.

The glutton's vilest enemy and greatest hazard is not deprivation but temptation. The two are related, but they are different nevertheless. If a glutton is locked up in jail, his eating will be greatly reduced both in quantity and quality by forces outside his control. He will then suffer real deprivation.


But that deprivation is not the same as the temptation that assails him when he is at liberty, virtually surrounded — it seems to him — by restaurants, delicatessens, markets, food stores and people of normal weight who eat the most delicious and fattening things from morning until night, and where all he has to do is "give in." In prison he cannot give in. This physical restraint obviates the agonizing conflict he suffers in liberty.


Put a drug addict in a hospital under lock and key, and even though he will suffer his "cold turkey" withdrawal, he will at least be spared the temptation of running out into the street to buy another "fix." But if he tries to go cold turkey on his own, he will not only have to suffer the withdrawal pangs, but also the temptation to forget his resolve to stay clean and go back on drugs to get some relief from his craving.

The glutton, too, though his deprivation gives him great discomforts when he curbs his appetite, is far more plagued by the temptation than the deprivation to give in and give up.

What is temptation? To tempt is a Latin-rooted word for "to try." Temptation is trial. The word trial, in turn, has several meanings. To try <u>something</u> is to do something one is not sure one can do, or whether one likes it. To try <u>someone</u> is to put him to the test. To be tried means that an attempt (trial) is made by someone, or by oneself, or by God, or by the devil, to see whether one can stand up to something difficult. Tempt-ation is an at-tempt made on us by some outside force, something we are being put through and better resist!

It is therefore wrong to say that some foods tempt us. That food is dumb and cannot tempt anybody. Something else or someone else (our ego) is tempting us, trying us, trying or testing the fortitude of our resolve, and triumphing if we give in.

In the case of food, it is not the food that is tempting or trying us, but that wily monster – gluttony. In the Middle Ages, all temptation was simply ascribed to the devil who was believed to be a scheming, living, powerful and destructive creature, luring his victims into perdition with things that seemed desirable and delicious but in reality were not. That the devil is an explanation for one's indulged weaknesses is much more comfortable as an excuse for our transgressions than to blame the "id" or whatever shibboleth we use in our day.

In his moments of temptation, the conflicted glutton should not regard his predicament as a battle between himself and a morsel of food, but rather as a temptation that originates somewhere else. He should see that he is tempted by powers outside himself plus that second helping; that he is tempted as by the devil — or tried by a jury.

In this an uneven struggle? Has he no allies in this battle? That is up to him. But if he remembers the "devilish" aspect of the tempt-ation, namely that to indulge it does not produce lasting satisfaction but gnawing remorse, he will be better equipped to confront the devil lurking in that dish, and overcome him. In fact, faced with an attractive dish of food, the glutton might try to make himself consciously aware of the fact that not the food but the devil himself is staring him in the face.

SEVENTEEN:  The glutton must learn how to dance.

This curious demand is meant both literally and figuratively. In the literal sense, the glutton often has a problem with dancing. Being overweight and vain, emotionally aggressive but physically timid, and therefore often clumsy and inhibited, i.e., "self" conscious in a dozen painful ways, he may avoid dancing even if he loves it. And in his mind he loves to dance.

One fine thing about dancing is that one cannot dance and be craving food at the same time. Even the confirmed glutton, if he has ever been on the floor at a dinner dance, knows that when he is moving to the music with a partner of the opposite sex – even if that partner holds no great attraction or interest for him – he is not his customarily voracious self. He does not even feel any particular urgency to return to his table to eat.

One reason for this seems to be that physical motion, and especially rhythmical motion, reduces one's appetite. Physical immobility, on the other hand, and the absence – or disturbance – of an inner or external rhythm or beat, stimulates it.

But it is hard for the glutton to dance, not just because he is so self-conscious. He is also anxious to remain in control. The dancer, even if he seems in control of the steps he is taking and that he makes his partner take, abandons himself to the music, the rhythm, the beat. While the music lasts he is "in tune" and "above food," so to speak. He dances. When the music stops, he returns to his "old" self. While dancing he temporarily gives up control and enjoys it.

He also enjoys — and is distracted by — the physical proximity and touch of another person (perhaps a stranger), a situation the glutton seems more eager to avoid than most. Thus the glutton should bring himself to dance. It will help him not only to reduce his gluttony, but also help him to become a person with less violent appetites. Beyond that, dancing in the figurative sense, as a mode of doing things, and of doing them with ease and panache, is another aim for which the glutton should strive.

Some people literally "dance" through life, with an ease and nimbleness most of us can only envy. For the fact is that most of us, especially the glutton, are plodders. We bulldoze, or try to bulldoze, our way through what we regard as a thicket of recalcitrant obstacles and of people who seem to stand in our way. And we do it grimly.

But the dancer is not grim while he is dancing. As dancing and grimness do not go together but grimness and gluttony do, the lesson is obvious. We might not just exhort the glutton to dance but dance a little more ourselves. In our current culture everybody, it seems, urges everybody else to "relax." This indicates that in our unrelaxed society to "relax" is at a real premium. We therefore envy those who "dance through life." And while we urge it on the glutton, we might try it ourselves.

**EIGHTEEN:   The glutton must learn to accept acceptance.**

Half a century ago the great theologian Paul Tillich ventured the thought that acceptance itself required some accepting from those who needed it. What does this mean, and how does it unfold?

In the context of gluttony, overeating is a silent rebellion against one's own life, its course and the state of the world in general, as one sees it. The overeater is generally not an acceptor. First and foremost among the things he does not accept is, of course, his weight and shape. Beyond that he does not accept his love life, his marriage, his work, his "friends," or the President of the United States. But his non-acceptance is mostly passive; he does not really do anything about the things or people that trouble him. The world that he tends to either mock with acerbic wit or malign takes little note of him.   And overeating results from all his frustrations.   And all his frustrations, in turn, are the result of his not accepting things as they are or as he has made them to be for himself. It is not just his weight and build he cannot accept, it also is his gnawing appetite, his sexual frustrations, his work, his role in the world. Beyond that, he cannot accept the rhythm of creation   —   the constant change, death, accidents, incidents, and man's lack of control over events. All this stimulates his passion for a juicy hamburger with a side order of fries.

To change over to a frame of mind and soul where his greed will abate, he must diminish his frustrations. This means he must become more realistic. He has to accept the ways of this world and society in it, and even the cards his fatum has dealt him. Verily it is better — and the glutton will find it so — to face reality, vexing though it may be, than to bury it under a bushel of gourmet food.

A random example might illuminate this opaque but important point. If I have a decrepit automobile that breaks down frequently, and I dream of tooling around in the new Ferrari I can't afford, I have a choice. I can dislike my old car, and, while riding in it, dream my frustrating dream of that Ferrari. Or I can have my old car repaired, buy new tires, and give it a new paint job. But I can only do the latter if and when I accept the old jalopy as my car. I must stop rejecting it. I must stop disliking it. I must accept it as mine, just as I must accept my home or job or life as mine before I can improve it. Perhaps eventually I can turn it into something different. But I must first accept it, and not with gritted teeth but with an accepting mind.

Similarly, if I want to attain a lower weight and keep it there, I must — aside from so many other things — first accept my body, and everything else about myself. Otherwise, I will never even begin to battle my frustrations, but remain in the sloth of inaction, abandoning myself to my gourmandizing..

But I must do this accepting of my reality without resentment, for accepting anything with resentment is always an acceptance with reservations. This in turn will stay my hand sooner or later in my efforts at changing.

Thus, only acceptance without resentment — even of what we had thought was unacceptable — is "accepting acceptance." Which means to accept, at first, everything we find when surveying our situation, and then accepting all that needs to be done to change it. First there must be acceptance of what we find.

One reason the glutton has such a hard time accepting anything is that the entire notion of acceptance is foreign and even repugnant to him. Instead he is a dreamer. He is even rebellious, although his rebellion is passive. And he tends to look down on people who accept their lot like so many lambs. But, paradoxically, he also looks down on those who strive to improve themselves and their lot. Thus he cannot have what he wants either way.

It is not suggested that the glutton accept himself as he is. We merely remind him that he must first accept himself as he is today and then accept that acceptance without rancor.

This is a *sine qua non* for his progress.

He must learn to see and accept himself as an acceptor of life as it is, and of the limitations of all he can do with it. And he will find that to first accept it is, in itself, a great relief. Every mourner eventually discovers this, once he accepts his loss. The glutton, too, will feel relief once he accepts the need for and benefits of acceptance.

Accepting acceptance can be seen in different ways. Friedrich Nietzsche said that the difference between the slave and the free man is that the slave's road through life follows the signpost: "You must!" whereas the free man's road through life is guided by: "I want!"

If there is truth in that, all the eighteen "Musts" given above are not things the glutton should feel he <u>has</u> to do, but should learn to <u>want</u>.

He then will become free, to the limited extent man can be free. And attainable freedom certainly includes freedom from slavery to food.

# CONCLUSION

**Well, there, that is all.**

**All? What, still no miracle diet? No panacea? No magic mantra the glutton, if he even read this far, has been secretly hoping for all along despite earlier warnings to the contrary?**

**Perhaps the glutton does not realize that he has been presented here with a detailed program and remedy against a great and tricky ill. If he penetrates with his mind what was said, and follows the suggestions, he will change his personality, lose his gluttony, and become a person of normal appetite, i.e., normal weight, without deprivation or diet.**

**And, wonder of wonders, he will even be able to enjoy his food _more_, since he will be able to savor it without feeling guilty. He will be able to eat without the greed which increases the desire but reduces the enjoyment.**

**He will no longer hate or despise himself. Therefore, he will no longer despite others. The contempt in which he has held so much and so many, as a  —  necessary  —**

means of self-defense, will abate and dwindle. He will become active where he was once passive, and creative where he was parasitical. He will be able to accept himself and many others. But he will no longer accept his gluttony (as opposed to the days when he did not accept himself or others but, albeit reluctantly, accepted his gluttony).

So, basta! The insights presented in this small book are based on the experiences of many sufferers, including the author's. If the reader should heed what lessons spring from what others have endured, he will not be disappointed.

I will leave the reader with two more thoughts:

One of the glutton's underpinnings is his excessive individualism. We make a great deal of the precious individualism in our Western world, and indeed that individualism distinguishes man from the animal roaming in a collective herd. But, like every good thing, individualism can be overdone. It then leads to feelings of loneliness and isolation on the one hand, and of insignificance and lack of social purpose on the other.

The demagogues of fascism know what is attractive about totalitarian collectivism: the tribal, mythical solidarity of everyone with every other member of the vast group, and some extra-individual purpose, and be it even such an absurdity as Hitler's planned Thousand Year Reich.

The average glutton has no such sustaining bonds of companionship nor compelling interests beyond his personal concerns. He tends to be a loner, rather than a true individualist. Of course, some people make out very well in their lonely isolation, but only those who are overly religious or perhaps an Albert Einstein. Such people may not believe in others but only in God. The glutton, not believing in either, is always a sort of apocalyptician, an *"après moi le dèluge"* man, which is one reason why he craves food so much; his food is a pacifier and a means to propitiate the vast and somber forces he feels are all arrayed against him.

The other thought with which I want to leave the over-eater is that he cannot "give up" and give in to his craving even if in his distress he would want to. Elsewhere in this book a yogi was quoted that a glutton "had given up on his life." That is correct as far as it goes, but it does not go all the way.

The — perhaps terrifying — fact is that, short of committing suicide, one cannot give up on life. One can give up many dreams to become a millionaire or a tennis star, or an irresistible person or find the secret sources of the Nile; and more often than not life will be the better at least for the ensuing effort.

But one cannot give up on life itself, as it keeps going on and reasserting itself. Even to drink oneself to death, because one is trying to give up on life, is very difficult. It takes years of agony, hangovers, madness and physical illness. To eat oneself to death is even harder. The glutton who decides in a moment of despair, be it over his life in general or his gluttony in particular, that the game is not worth the candle and that he may as well eat forever all he wants never gets very far with this ignoble decision.

He always "comes to" again, only fatter and with more valuable time irretrievable wasted; and he is always confronted again with the arduous task to get himself back in hand. Why, then, should he not learn to make an easy habit of finally relegating food where it belongs: a great and unique pleasure that is altogether painless for those who have learned to "live" with it.

## Postscriptum

The reader will be surprised to find our treatise on gluttony concluding with words by Dwight D. Eisenhower, a man who, except for a "great steak," had no particular interest in food and least of all in feasting. Any overeater would do well to take his three favorite precepts to heart – precepts he stated often and that were validated by his own great successes:

**ROME WAS NOT BUILT IN A DAY**

**YOU CAN'T TEACH A DOG RELIGION**

**YOUR JOB – NOT YOU – IS IMPORTANT**

Taken together, these three precepts are a useful mantra for all gluttons, even though they say nothing about food or eating or gluttony or overweight or dieting or carbohydrates or waistlines or body fat or any of the things gluttons are constantly considering, studying, weighing, talking about, worrying about, observing and – violating.

The three precepts, or homilies, say all the glutton must observe if he wants to learn how to become the master and not the servant of his/her vice. They mean:

1. Anything worth doing takes time, often a long time, i.e., *patience.*

2. You can do only what can be done, not what man cannot do.

3. You must get off *your* self and devote *your* self to other things.

No better advice can be given to the glutton who is morbidly impatient, full to unreachable fantasies, and egocentric rather than concerned with other persons or things.

Any overeater or overcraver of food can cure him/herself *in time,* of his/her affliction, and *enjoy* food AND have a desirable weight – and maintain it *without* effort or diet until the day he/she dies. But haste – as in *any* quick diet – makes waste. *All* diets are painful and unproductive in the long run. This is a body blow to the glutton who is invariably also a dieter; he is as addicted to diets as he is to food. He even talks about "his" diet with fellow gluttons with the same intensity as he talks with them about, say, a brand new dish prepared by the incomparable Paul Prudhomme in his incomparable New Orleans temple where serious gourmets congregate to pay obeisance to their demanding palates.

But by "thinking right" the glutton can come to believe in his *gut* (pardon the joke!) that we do not live to eat but . . . and throw off his yoke! That is, if he can re-form his thinking and feeling about food and himself.